WITHDRAWN

THE
WARDROBE
WAKEUP

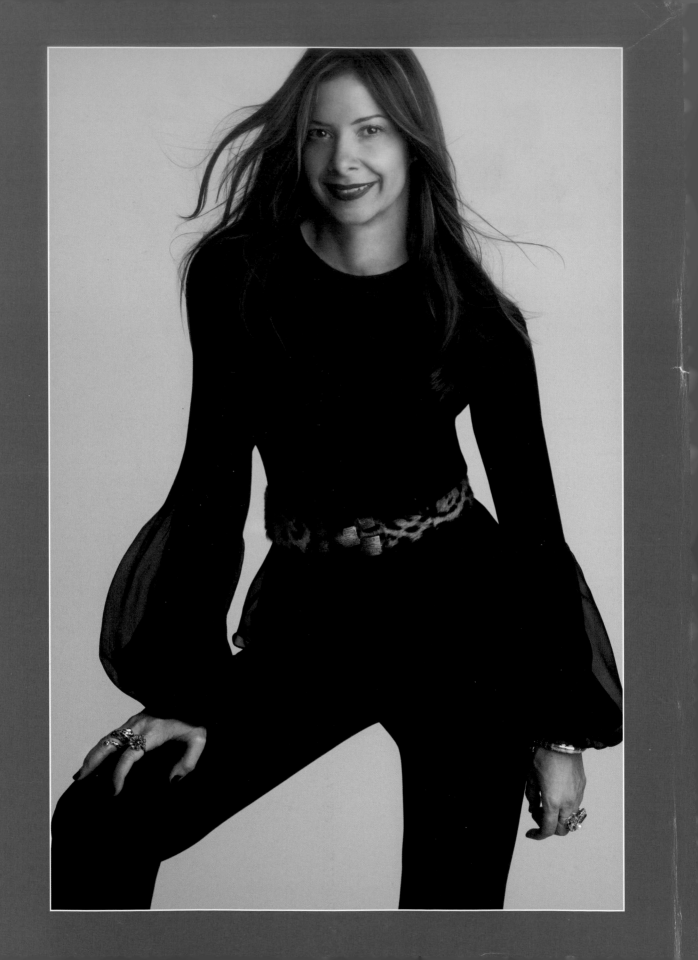

THE WARDROBE WAKEUP

Your Guide to Looking Fabulous at Any Age

LOIS JOY JOHNSON

Photography by
MICHAEL WARING

Foreword by
CHERYL TIEGS

Running Press
PHILADELPHIA · LONDON

© 2012 by Lois Joy Johnson
Photography © Michael Waring
Published by Running Press,
A Member of the Perseus Books Group

Books published by Running Press are available at special discounts for bulk purchases in the United States by corporations, institutions, and other organizations. For more information, please contact the Special Markets Department at the Perseus Books Group, 2300 Chestnut Street, Suite 200, Philadelphia, PA 19103, or call (800) 810-4145, ext. 5000, or e-mail special.markets@perseusbooks.com.

ISBN 978-0-7624-4584-4
Library of Congress Control Number: 2012947344

E-book ISBN 978-0-7624-4692-6

9   8   7   6   5   4   3   2   1
Digit on the right indicates the number of this printing

Designed by Corinda Cook
Edited by Cindy De La Hoz
Typography: Avenir, Aviano, Baskerville, Bodoni, Flama, and Helvetica Neue

Running Press Book Publishers
2300 Chestnut Street
Philadelphia, PA 19103-4371

Visit us on the web!
www.runningpress.com

To my BFFs, the girlfriends
who have always been there
for me 365 days a year, 24/7!

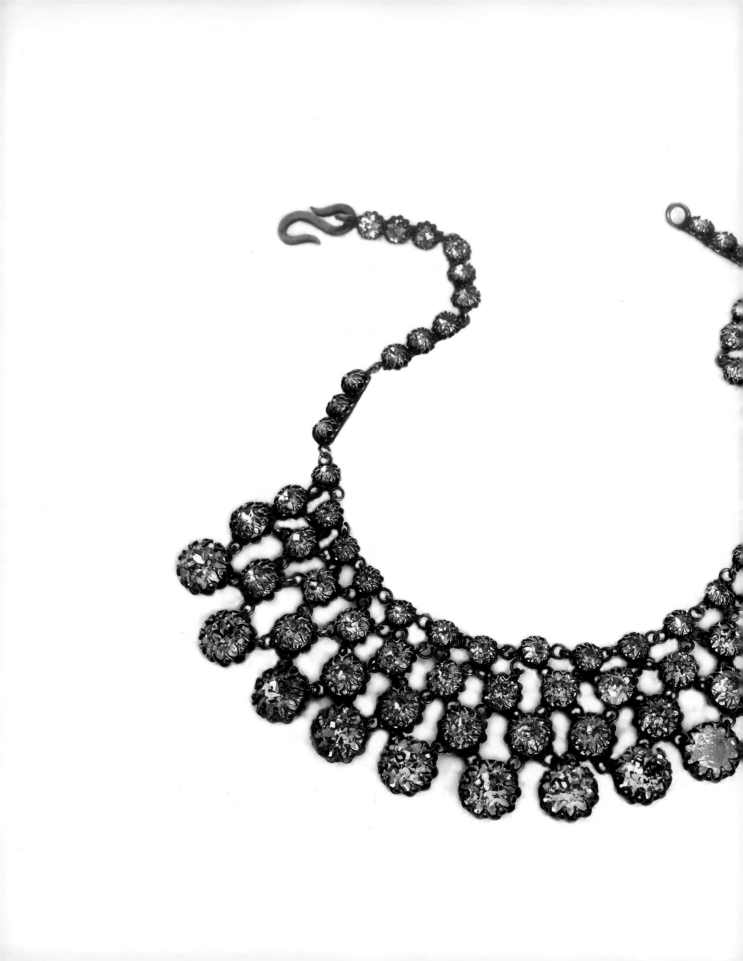

CONTENTS

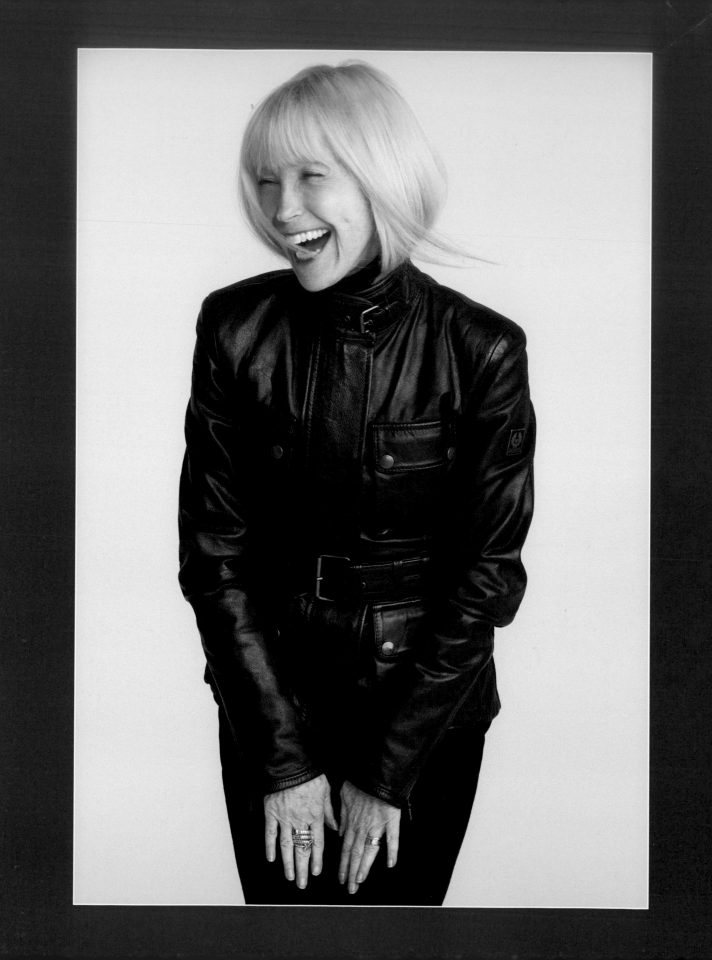

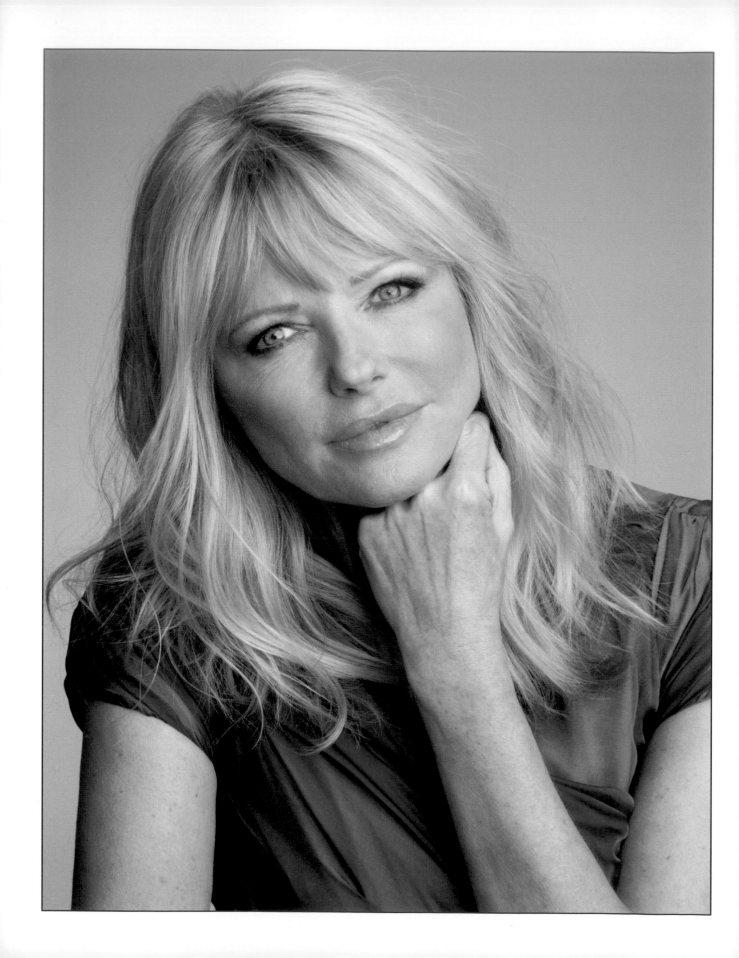

Life Is a Dressy Occasion: How To Get It Right

Once upon a time I was a happy, healthy California girl with five dresses hanging in my closet . . . one for each day of the high school week. It fit my lifestyle and I was content. Then I got a phone call from *Glamour* magazine in New York. They booked me to go down to St. Thomas in the Virgin Islands for a photo shoot. So I took a light yellow dress from my closet and thought it would make the cut. When the group decided to go out to dinner and a nightclub I realized my wardrobe was sorely lacking. I will always be grateful to the other model on the job, Ali MacGraw, who opened her suitcase and threw dress after dress (each with the tags still on) across the room for me to wear. Her generosity was and will always be much appreciated.

That's when I realized I had to put some thought into my wardrobe. If I was going to travel the world and work in all kinds of different climates I had better be prepared. So I came up with a system that still works for me to this day. I decided what my core items would be: well-cut pants in different fabrics; one-of-a-kind silk shirts; T-shirts; tailored skirts and blazers; sweaters in subtle colors; cool jackets; and coats. I always prefer to put on one outfit that will get me through the whole day and classic styles to offbeat zany ones. Coming up with a really successful offbeat look takes a lot of time, thought, and creativity, and unless you get it exactly right it usually comes out exactly wrong.

Whatever fashion imagination I have blossoms at night, when I put some real effort and ingenuity into the way I dress. I love the fantasy of evening clothes—shiny fabrics; satins; velvets; rhinestone belts; and sexy, strappy sandals. One of my favorite outfits for evening is a pair of tight turquoise jeans that I wear with my brilliant purple faux fox fur.

I'm fortunate enough to have worked often with Lois Joy Johnson—you should be so lucky! She had the great instinct to intuit who I was and how I would feel comfortable. She wouldn't insist I wear a trendy look for a shoot. We would go through racks of clothes and decide which ones fit my personality. And the whole time we had fun and a lot of laughs!

Find a mentor for yourself. If you know a beautifully dressed woman, someone whose fashion sense you admire, watch what she wears, notice how she combines colors and fabrics, how she puts her clothes together, and how she uses jewelry, belts, and scarves to create her own style. You don't need to copy what she's wearing but be open to ideas and inspiration.

I could go on and on but I think it's time for you to turn the page and read. There is a treasure trove of inspiration in this book. Lois Joy Johnson has made sense of this wonderful wide world of fashion. Enjoy!

—Cheryl Tiegs

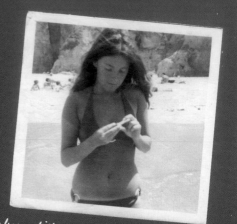

Baby editor me on a beach shoot

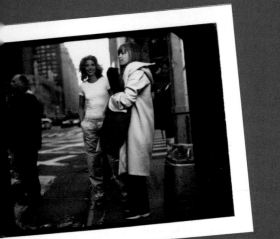

On an NYC street shoot
with Candace Bushnell

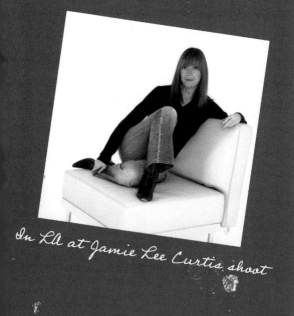

In LA at Jamie Lee Curtis shoot

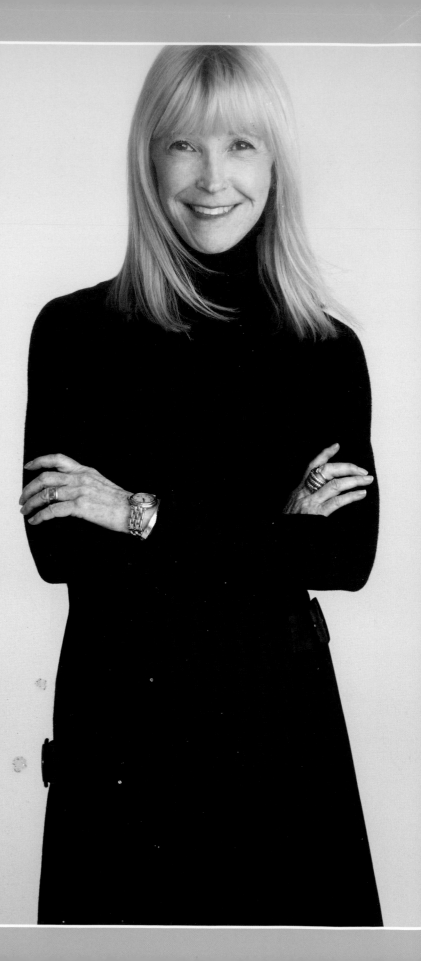

THE WARDROBE WAKEUP

INTRODUCTION BY LOIS JOY JOHNSON

After a certain age women and their clothes just don't get along anymore.

The romance is over. The body you've dressed and shopped for has evolved but your wardrobe hasn't. Clothes and looks that made you feel sexier, more confident, successful, well-dressed, and put together in your twenties, thirties, and early forties suddenly don't do it for you anymore. Changes in weight, hormones, work, finances, lifestyle, attitudes, opinions, and needs have had a major impact on your closet and style.

As a top fashion editor (and one of the founding editors of *MORE* magazine, where I was beauty and fashion director from 1998 to 2008), I've spent twenty plus years working with thousands of my readers and A-list models and celebrities to redefine how women dress after forty. I've also interviewed and photographed hundreds of women who changed forever the way we dress, shop, and think about clothes, including

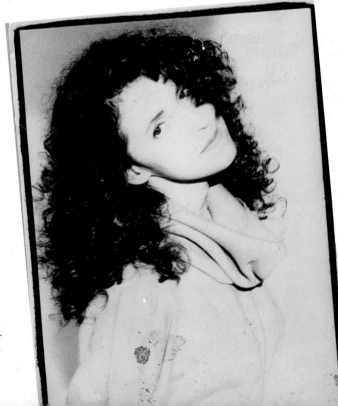

Taken by Francesco Scavullo in 1985: Me with brunette curls and cowl-neck cashmere

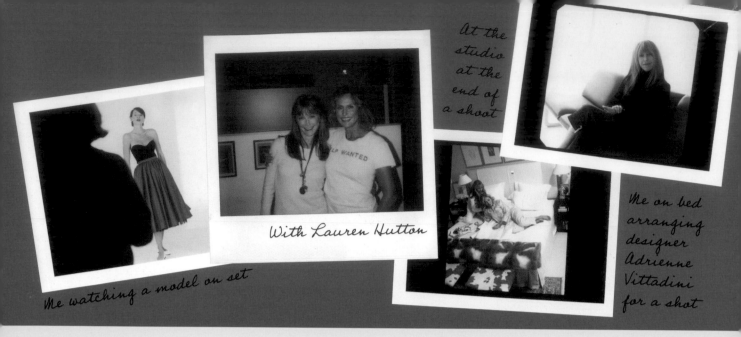

At the studio at the end of a shoot

With Lauren Hutton

Me on bed arranging designer Adrienne Vittadini for a shot

Me watching a model on set

Diane Keaton, Diane von Furstenberg, Cheryl Tiegs, and Lauren Hutton. Like you, I've griped about age, sag, flab, the high price of good clothes, the things I can't wear anymore, and those that I do.

The Wardrobe Wakeup is a realistic, honest fashion guide that crunches all my experience and knowledge into practical lessons and tips. You'll learn hundreds of body-enhancing, style-boosting, closet-reviving, money-saving tricks—straight from a fashion editor's mouth. It will give you the practical, chic strategies that do work for your everyday life starting right now.

In this book you'll also meet eighteen extraordinary women that are highlighted throughout—each remarkable in her own way and a fashion pro in her own right. All have survived trends, fads of the minute, weight changes, husbands, jobs, grown-up kids, and life's little lemons with wit and style. Find yourself in them, or maybe like me you'll be a combo.

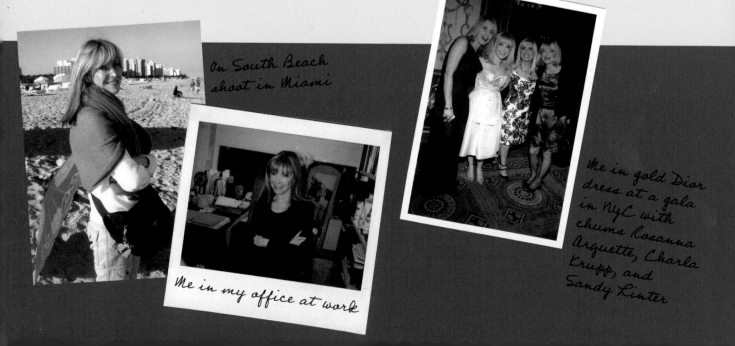

On South Beach shoot in Miami

Me in gold Dior dress at a gala in NYC with chums Rosanna Arquette, Charla Krupp, and Sandy Linter

Me in my office at work

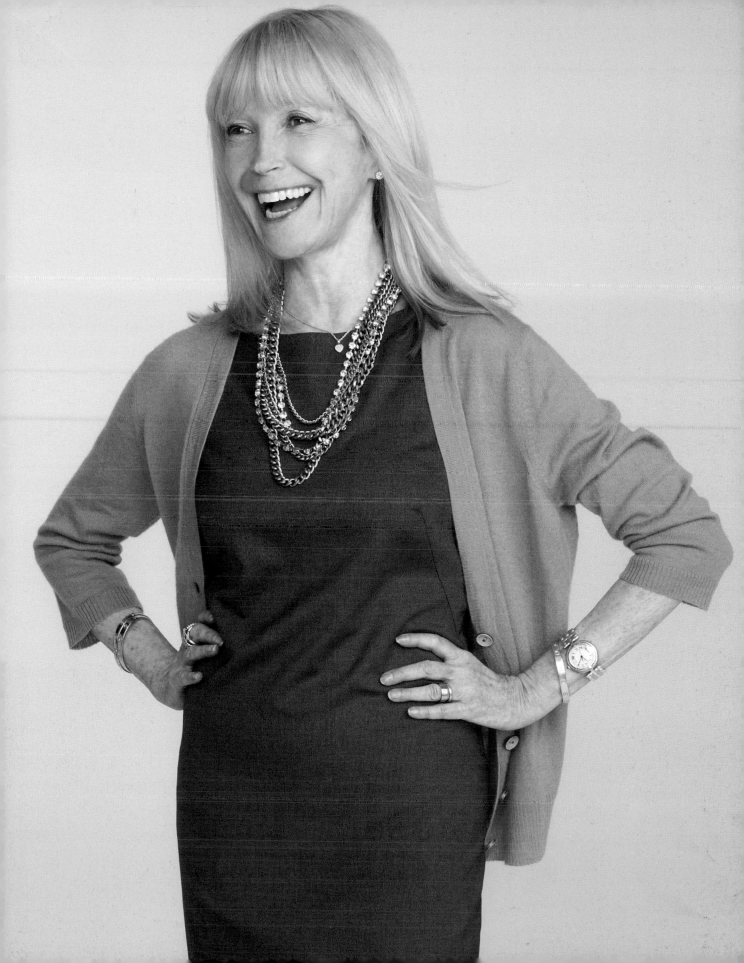

Use this book three ways.

1 **If you want more style and flattery from your same old clothes—without having to buy a thing (okay, maybe one or two things, but honestly that's it!).** The tricks I relied on as a fashion editor can update everything in your closet, de-age your look, and slim you down. For some women this is good enough. You'll learn to layer like a stylist, mix prints and colors like top designers do, and restore "lazy" clothes to activewear again. Find out exactly which sweaters, pants, skirts, and tops are the only ones worth keeping before you let them go.

2 **If you want to look contemporary but not silly, spend less but look better, and dress for comfort without giving up on fashion.** I'm going to let you in on the pro secrets to wearing leggings and jeans, how to really tie a scarf and a pareo, the one best pant style to buy, how to make low-cost clothes look like couture, how to give up stilettos and tight or skin-revealing clothes without losing your shape or sex appeal, why dresses and prints are always the best bets, the cheap deals to never pass up again, and where to find smart fashion now.

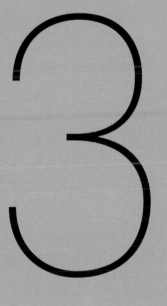

If you're starting over after a major lifestyle transition, financial change, job loss, weight change, or divorce. I'll tell you what to wear for the job interview when the competition is age thirty-five, how to dress when dating a much younger or much older man, or if you're going back to college. Find out how to look slim and stylish for a college reunion or your second wedding. Learn when to wear sheer panty-hose and when to go barelegged, what to wear on a cruise, a long road trip, to your kid's engagement party or when you finally meet his ex and family. **You'll look fresher, hipper, and hotter than ever and your clothes will, too.**

CHAPTER ONE

SAME OLD CLOTHES, 10X MORE STYLE!

Clothes are a necessity, fashion is an option, and style is your choice.

Whether your very chic satchel bag is a $59 faux leather bargain from Target, a $398 leather classic from Coach, or a $1,950 pebbled leather splurge from Salvatore Ferragamo, you control the purse strings for trillions of dollars and most of the financial wealth in the U.S. As babes-of-a-certain-age we're the largest, richest, smartest segment of the population, with more spending clout than any other group. In fact, we're the real wizards behind the Oz-es of the fashion industry. We've "made" designers, set trends, and practically invented the dress-down look everyone now calls "lifestyle clothes." We're informed, opinionated, and super-savvy about sales and bargains. We know our H&M from our Hermès, our Gap from our Gucci, and our Banana Republic from our Burberry. But when it comes to clothes, our relationship goes way beyond money, trends, and the runway—it's emotional. We used to dress to fit in, stand out, or move up. Now we dress only for ourselves . . . at least that's our line and we're sticking to it!

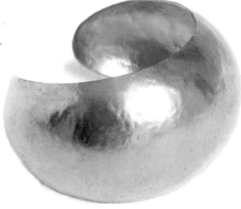

Here's the real backstory

Your closet, like mine, is probably a compilation of past and present, designer labels and cheapie finds, good buys and bad choices, sweet memories of good times and some difficult ones too. And you probably have more stuff than you really need.

We all have keepers—the clothes that were our allies. They made us

feel fashionable, sexy, thin, comfortable, confident, successful, well-dressed, and/or put-together. They helped us juggle kids and careers, relationships and schedules, hormones and diets, and we're so grateful they did. We owe them.

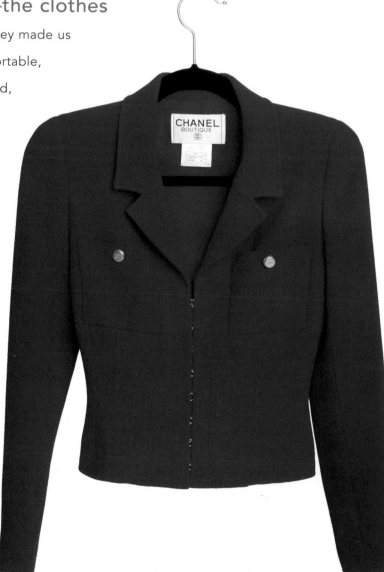

Q

- No new clothes?
- What's YOUR reason?

A

Guilt. Money. New priorities. Fashion's gotten too hard to deal with. Some of us refuse to buy new clothes. We're done . . . at least for now.

The reasons are diverse. New financial concerns or business projects come first. Passions like travel, gardening, and home renovation are getting more of our attention. Social consciousness and environmental concerns make us want to minimize the clutter, even in our closets. Lots of women feel they have enough clothes and don't have a need to buy more of the same. Major lifestyle switches or work changes for many have brought lifetime shopping habits to a screeching halt. Some women say fashion itself is to blame. They think it's gotten too young, too hard-to-wear, too trendy, or just too expensive.

One thing's for sure: our bodies change, sag, and shift whether our weight goes up, down, or stays the same. Yet many of us say we're in the best shape of our lives and appreciate or at least accept our bodies more. We eat healthier, work out, feel stronger, energized, and more toned. We're more in control of the way we look than we were at 25. This is a huge influence on what we buy and wear.

What a wardrobe shake-up can do for you now

This chapter is a friendly fashion intervention for grown-up women with a past. It's devoted to those of us with new lives, evolving bodies, fresh attitudes, and the same old clothes. Stay the course because fashion is 50 percent clothes and 50 percent hocus-pocus.

Styling tricks make clothes work, not the clothes themselves.

We all benefit from a little deception and cheating. Illusion is part of every fashion photo or store display you see. It's behind every well-dressed woman on the street or magazine ad, and simmers beneath every runway show. The job of a good fashion editor or stylist is to make anything—no matter how boring, baggy, cheap, weirdly colored, oddly patterned, or unappealing—look great, desirable, and most of all wearable. Simply by manipulating color and proportion you can update, slim down, and get more versatility from your same clothes. Don't let them sit in the closet.

We're not our mothers (in truth we're not even like our old selves ten years ago). We don't buy clothes for perpetuity. I've given up minis, chunky sweaters, and big dangly earrings forever. Your turn!

Remember: If you don't wear it, it doesn't count.

Me too! Same thing! A few years ago my whole life changed. I went from a glam big-city magazine career to working from home as a freelance editor/columnist/author. My new daily routine in the suburbs did not require fresh pairs of Manolos and seasonal updates of designer duds. Jeans, ballet flats, boots, and layers of tees under sweaters became my new year-round "uniform." This was huge. I'd put in decades as a fashion editor, sitting front row at major fashion shows. My days were all about market appointments, pre-shoot run throughs, designer look books, and the photo shoots that followed. I'd spent years dressing and styling thousands of women in their forties, fifties, and sixties for magazine photos and covers. Then the unexpected happened. Add my new at-home gig and dress-down lifestyle to a post-menopause body, a fresh frugality towards shopping, and a move from a house to an apartment with less closet space, and you get the idea. I gave away my bikinis, hid my Amex, and bought my first pair of SPANX.

Lois in her daily jeans uniform

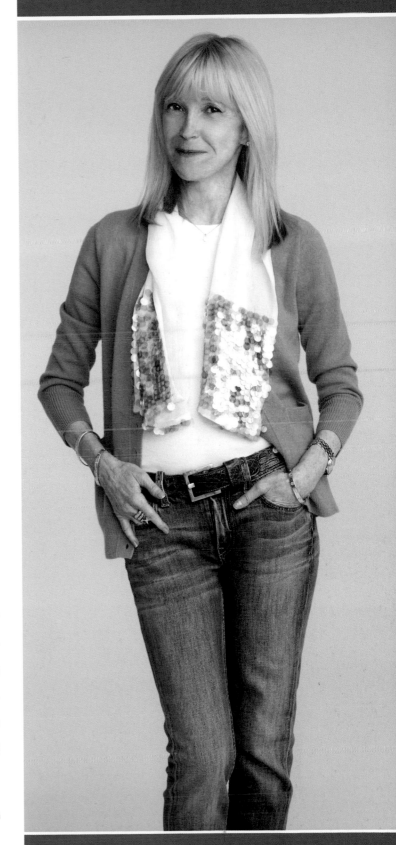

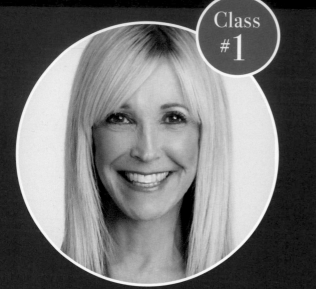

Class #1

10 Big Tricks To Teach Your Same Old Clothes

You don't need to buy a thing to make these tricks work for you. However, let's be realistic. One or two items you don't have just might turn your entire closet around, so never say never. I bet you think I'm going to start by saying, "wear black." There isn't one woman over forty who doesn't believe black makes her look thinner. Good luck with that because if your black clothes are oversized, boxy, shapeless, too tight, too short, or too shiny . . . they won't work for you now. This doesn't mean stop wearing so much black. It still makes us feel sophisticated, glam, and cool. But to tell you the truth, now that everyone from baristas to girls in junior high to toddlers wear black, the edge is dulled. We need new ways to rekindle the attraction and a lot more options. Start with your closet.

1. Edit . . . just like an A-list store.

Turn your closet into a curated, edited collection instead of a hit-or-miss jumble. Fashion directors of fancy department stores say their merchandise is "curated." This means the clothes were tastefully and carefully selected above and beyond the usual humdrum process. Magazine editors—especially old school ones like me—use the term "edited" instead, to describe the ultimate fashion options selected at run-throughs, that get to go on to the studio or location for the final shoot. Let both terms inspire you to weed out the trash and start working your own racks with a plan. Anything beyond rejuvenation—frayed, pilled, stiff, too mini, too clingy, way too big, too saggy, or small—out! Yes, even if it's black and even if it has a big-deal designer label. Those fifteen pairs of jeans you don't wear? Toss them, too.

Organize what's left by color—all your black items together, all your navy things, all your browns, all your oranges, blah blah.

Don't get obsessive about exact shade, fabric, or season. Within each color grouping there will be a range of tones from dark to light, differences in fabrics and textures, plain and fancy, solids and prints, super-casual and dressy, and tailored and relaxed. Organize prints, florals, and stripes according to their dominant color. Fold and stack sweaters, tees, knits, and tanks by color and arrange shoes, belts, and bags by color as well. This system makes layering and accessorizing easy, increases your mixing options, and cuts dressing time in half.

Next, hang like items together within each color group. Cluster jackets, tops, pants, jeans, skirts, and dresses within each color section.

2. Wear one color
head-to-toe. It's a style home run.

Big-time designers like Michael Kors, Ralph Lauren, Donna Karan, Giorgio Armani, and Eileen Fisher often use the one-color strategy of dressing (also called "tonal dressing") in their collections. Pairing tops and bottoms in the same color is a quick, fool-proof formula for style. What-goes-with-what is never an issue and you always look longer and slimmer. Your new closet set-up makes it easy.

I know it's tempting to wear black pants with a crisp white shirt or a red sweater with your jeans but breaking the line of your body at the waist or hip with a sharp color contrast is never going to be your slimmest option.

An exact, or rather almost exact, match top and bottom gives you the slimmest look of all. Be realistic though; unless you stick to wearing just pieces from the same designer, same fabric, and same year dye lot (and that's just not possible for 99 percent of us), a true color match top and bottom is not a reality, so don't drive yourself mad. You could "match" a navy wool sweater and dark blue jeans or a black cotton top with black cords. Even if you opt to just stay within the same color group you'll still get a sleeker vertical line.

Marilyn Glass in gray
agnès b., head to toe

3. Wear black with navy, like fashion editors do.

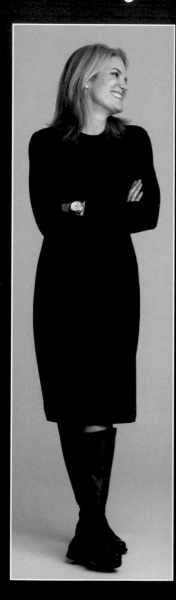

What if you like slimming benefits but don't want a "tough love," one-color approach every day? What if you don't have enough clothes in your individual color groups for plenty of one-color options? What if you've simply had it up to here with matchy-matchy? There's a foolproof color trick editors and designers use: pair two different colors of the same intensity—the same degree of darkness, lightness, or brightness. You don't want dramatic contrast. Good examples are black with navy, black with chocolate brown, charcoal or brown with burgundy. Neither color jumps out as being significantly lighter or brighter.

Start with accessories. Try brown shoes and a brown bag with a navy or black outfit. These color combos are favorites of French and Italian couture designers like Yves Saint Laurent and Giorgio Armani. Don't limit yourself to dark colors. Light, bright, or muted colors of the same intensity team up this way too. White with sand (a Ralph Lauren favorite), mustard with butterscotch, and rose with coral are a few ideas.

How to tell if your color combo works?

Squint at yourself in a full-length mirror. The transition from color to color should flow without an obvious sharp break where the two meet.

Jane Larkworthy

4. A longer neck and legs are game changers.

Get them.

Create the illusion of a swan-like neck and lanky legs by stretching your body at opposite ends with nude pumps and low-ish necklines that expose your upper chest. Anything you wear from now on can benefit from these two tips. Shoes that match your skin add inches to your legs even if you're 5'2". If you don't already own a pair, nude pumps are *the* reason to break your no-shopping rule.

Buy nude pumps in a skin-tone shade similar to your foundation makeup (sand, caramel, tan, or bronze, for example) in any heel height you prefer. Keep the toe tapered to get the maximum stretching and slimming effect.

You'll even get leg-lengthening benefits from skin-tone flats (these are amazing in summer with bare legs or cropped pants) or slim, nude knee-high boots (wear them with nude fishnets too in cold weather).

Next, "elongate" your neck with necklines that dip below your collarbones. Make these your first choice whenever possible. You don't need very low-cut necklines to get neck-stretching benefits, which is why I specify "low-ish." In fact, if you go too low and reveal cleavage it can sabotage the whole mission. Cowls, scoop, V-necks, and any shirt unbuttoned to form a V, work just fine.

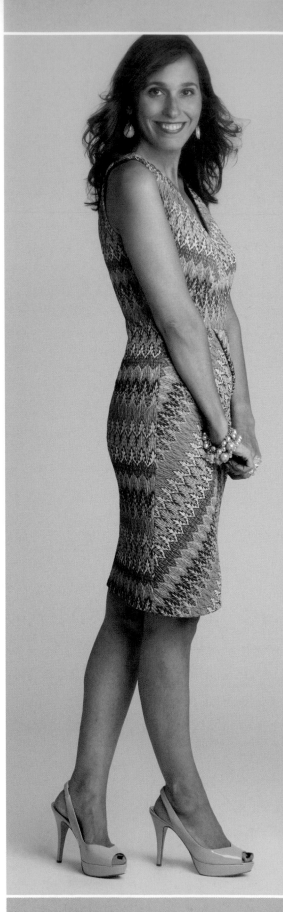

Hilary Black in V-neck print dress and nude shoes: neck and leg extenders

5. A nip and tuck freshens everything. A lift is essential after 40, but I mean the tailoring kind.

When samples arrive at a photo shoot they get a backstage tweak by an expert seamstress or tailor. Refining, enhancing, or exaggerating (in some cases) the fit of the clothes makes them look better in photos. Your own clothes can look newer, fit better, and become more wearable with the help of a tailor, too. It's a worthwhile expense if you want to really make use of what you own and look contemporary. **Here's how to revive your own wardrobe with photo shoot tailoring tricks:**

JACKETS: Deconstruct your boxy blazers and suit jackets. Get rid of the shoulder pads, and raise the shoulder line. By removing the pads and taking in the resulting excess fabric you instantly contemporize the entire jacket. Have your tailor raise the shoulder line, from neck to shoulder joint, for a smoother fit across the front. This prevents the fabric from buckling and creasing across the chest when you sit (a pet peeve of women with full busts). Shoulders should not extend past your own (no matter what the trend-of-the-minute is on runways), so don't get talked into reducing them only slightly. Ask your tailor to slim down the sleeves too. This raises the armhole and gives your arms and bust a firmer, more sculpted look.

A fitted jacket with a nipped waist will always make you feel and appear thinner so take in roomy or straight-cut jackets at the sides. It stretches the entire body by creating a longer illusion from the waist to toes. This is a must-do trick if, like me, you're on the short side.

SKIRTS: **Lower or remove the waist-band on all your old skirts.** This will add extra space between your bosom and waist, restore definition, and elongate your midriff. Everyone benefits but if you have a short torso and full bosom this step is really crucial. Have your tailor taper classic straight skirts to a slightly contoured pencil for a slimmer, more updated look. Before signing off on the tailoring job, test the skirts as pinned for ease and comfort. Try sitting, crossing your legs, and walking briskly. You don't want to go too tight or too pegged either.

Keep your skirts at a knee-grazing length (although the exact length will vary according to your legs and personal preference). The shortest you should go now is top of the knees or an inch or two above. The longest you should go is mid-knee, or just to the bottom of the kneecap.

PANTS: Old pants are a tricky call when it comes to alterations. New styles with improved proportions, design details, and body-friendly fabric blends have solved a lot of pants issues. Oldies hanging around our closets usually suffer from a poor fit or former-body syndrome. Ditch them and start fresh.

Here's the one tailoring exception for pants: if the overall pant shape is slim, the fit is smooth across your middle, and the fabric is excellent, alterations may be possible and worthwhile.

And keep your pants pockets open. Fashion pros suggest sewing pants pockets (and those on jackets) closed for a slimmer line, but I disagree. I think using pockets helps your body language and posture more than it hurts the look.

DRESSES: Tailoring makes sleeveless dresses more wearable. Even slight alterations at the bust, waist, and hip compensate for age and body changes. **To get a smoother line in front, take a dress in at the seams and raise the shoulder line.** This nip also tightens the armholes so your arms appear slimmer. Consider having a tailor modify high necks to wide shallow V or boat necks. Crop long evening gowns to the knees, and crop dressy minis into tunics.

COATS: **De-age your coats and rejuvenate the shape with snips at the sleeves and hem where they show wear.** Remove shoulder pads and trim excess fabric at the shoulders.

Hilary Black

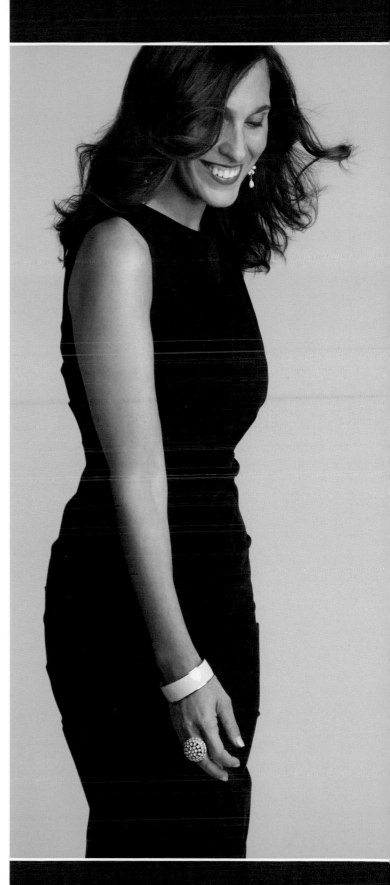

6. Layer your clothes like a stylist.

Layering gives all your clothes, but especially your casual pieces, a contemporary look. It updates the way you usually put looks together. Hipsters, teens, and French style icon Jane Birkin layer instinctively and almost better than anyone. To get the slouchy, cool effect, keep a sense of your body under layers at all times. Comfy layers get sloppy and "fat" fast if you don't.

The weight of the fabric and length of the item matter, so here's how you do it:

1. Layer your top half in this order:
Thinnest fabric to thickest from the inside out, longest layer first, and shortest last.

2. Start with a long tank.
A tank gives you a sleek base and bridges gaps at the waist. Unlike T-shirts, tanks won't add excess fabric around the shoulders and upper arms that can bulk up your shape as you layer. Fitted tanks look better under button-up shirts or slouchy, relaxed sweaters. Looser relaxed tanks look better under tailored jackets, where their body-skimming ease offsets the structured shape.

3. Add a V, ballet, or boat-neck tee and/or a shirt or blouse.
Any open, bare neckline is best to keep your neck long and visible.

4. Add a sweater, cardigan, or jacket.
Uneven lengths allow the layers to show.

5. Add a slim or relaxed piece on bottom.
You have two choices: pair layers with super-slim base, like leggings, fitted jeans, or slim ankle cropped pants. Or wear them with relaxed jeans, cargos, or khakis.

6. If you do a relaxed pant, define the waist with a belt.
Without showing definition at the waist, layers and a loose pant look dumpy. Choose a blazer or a long V cardigan as your top layer and wear it open to provide a peek at the belt you're wearing.

7. Let it all hang out.
Imperfection is important.

Let go of perfection. It's the little off details that make old clothes look stylish. The minute you start wearing your basics in a pristine way (buttoning shirts straight up to the neck, neatly matching turned back cuffs or tucking in tops cleanly), it's over. Your clothes will look dated and so will you. Instead, let long tanks, tops, and shirts dangle in plain sight beneath sweaters and jackets. Master the half-tuck. This means partially tucking in tanks or tops at the front and leaving them loose the rest of the way around you. Allow tanks and relaxed tees to drift in wide V or scoop necklines. Casually roll cuffs on shirts and jeans in an irregular way.

Loosen up. The giveaway may be a shirttail, tee hem, or tank strap showing bits of your layering in an obvious way. This is precisely what gives your same old clothes a more modern spin.

FYI, there's a chic fashion trick to rolling pants or boyfriend jeans at the bottom. First of all, only roll soft casual pants that have a broken-in look. Instead of folding the hem in neat flat cuffs, roll it to just above the anklebone, keeping the roll about an inch wide. That hint of ankle (a slim body zone, like wrists) helps to elongate the leg even if you're wearing flats. Pumps add a sexy, feminine spark but low kitten heels or jeweled flats stylishly contrast with boyish layers and rolled pants, too.

8. Wear your belts.
Skinny ones shape up every body.

Dig out all your belts, but especially narrow ones in the half- to one-inch range. Get them back in rotation and around your waist ASAP. They restore definition to your body and give structured clothes a stronger, more contemporary shape—so even tailored jackets and coats look new. Black, brown, and neutral beige leather in a range of textures work with everything. Super-skinny styles won't crowd your torso and they flatter every woman who thinks she can't or shouldn't wear belts. Include vintage chain belts in this category. They're adjustable (to accommodate anything from silk blouses to jackets) and the shot of gold or silver glams up your outfit.

One slim belt is all you need to refresh structured dresses, to feminize tailored jackets and suits, or to give flat-knit sweaters worn over skirts or pants a hint of shape.

Be sure to wear these belts at your waist and not your hip (where they are useless). Use them to sneak in a trendy touch—for example, patent, a bow, metallic finishes, or a pop of color. Wide corset belts and elaborate contoured styles are "statement" accessories and not for everyone. They take up a lot of midriff space, but if you have a long, slim torso with room to spare between your chest and waist, go for it. When it comes to your older hipster belts, slip those through the loops of your softest vintage jeans and wear them casually, even those with showy buckles.

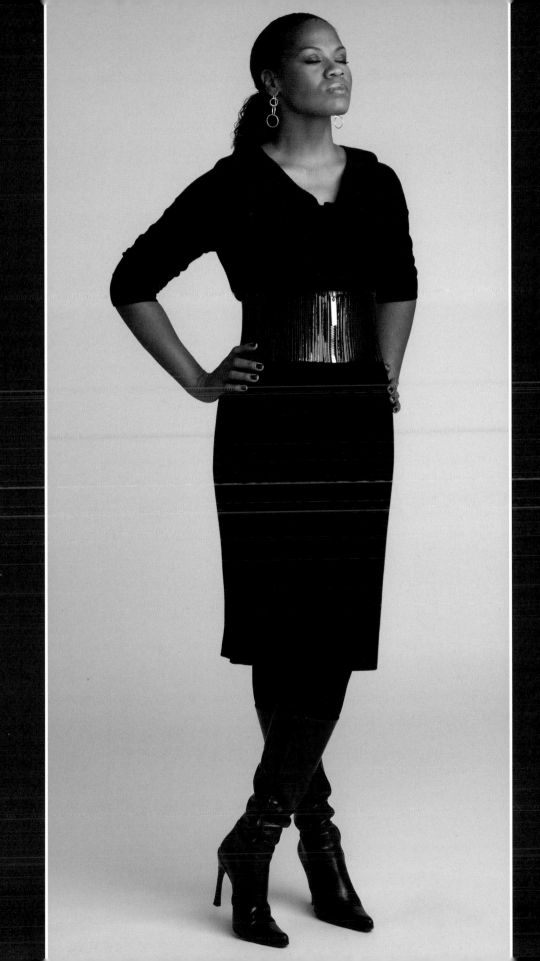

Cynde Watson

9. Mix prints to create new combos in seconds.

Combining two or more prints can give your wardrobe a new spin, but there's a catch. Clashing combos look great in fashion photos or when pre-mixed by designers, but for real life and real bodies there's only one way to pull it off without looking ridiculous.

Choose one color theme at a time. Something has to hold mixed prints together and color is a foolproof hook.

First, select one color group and pull out the print tops and bottoms. Include florals, tweeds, stripes, abstracts, geometrics, animal prints—anything in a pattern or menswear fabric. These will provide your potential combos. Pair print tops and bottoms. **If you're not used to clashing prints adding a third solid piece in the common color can make the look hang together more easily for you.** Let's say you lock in brown as your common color. You might pair a brown dotted silk blouse with an artsy brown graphic print skirt and throw on a brown cardigan to help it "gel."

Subtle or small-scale prints are easier to work with than large dramatic ones and won't look choppy, even on a petite frame. Designers recycle mixed prints as a "new trend" almost every year.

10. Wear status jewelry and accessories ironically.

Young stylists will do anything to get their hands on your old logo loaded and branded vintage accessories. These items still have style but need to be worn now with a breezy, low-key attitude. This way your Fendi baguettes, Chanel bags, and silver Tiffany chain-link bracelets can keep going forever. Just wear them with basics and sporty, low-cost clothes.

Use vintage bags, scarves, costume and real jewelry to punctuate casual clothes with a sense of your own personal fashion history . . . the older the better!

Add wit and personality by swapping your trench belt for an Hermès silk scarf. Snap sparkly clip-on earrings on plain ballet flats. Wear one big white pearl stud earring and one black. Twist ropes of pearls, chains, and ribbons together for a new chunky statement necklace. Just select one focal point at a time. You don't want to hit neck, wrists, and ears all at once like a Christmas tree.

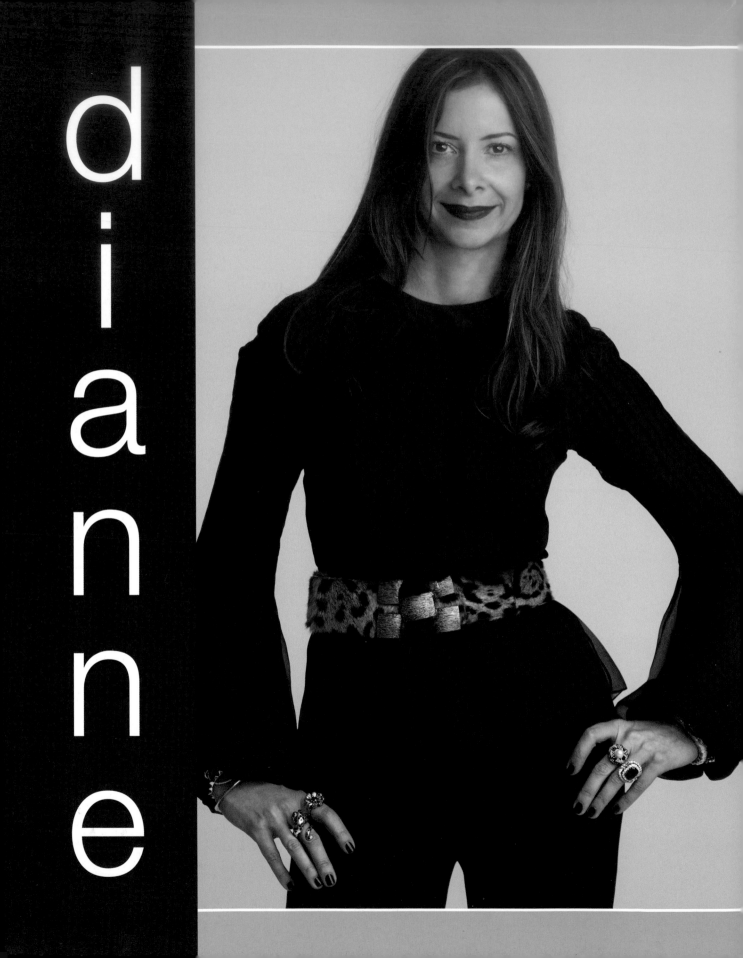

diane

dianne on:

style: "Being a full-time working, commuting mom-on-the-go, my personal style requires a mix of comfort and ease of transformation. I invest in iconic pieces that serve as my base and add in fun from the waist up—a great belt, vintage jewelry, or a chic bag. I wake up at the crack of dawn when it's still dark out and get ready before I wake my kids. My 'base' items get the most wear. They are all black: skinny jeans, pencil skirt, and wide-leg trousers."

inspiration: "Being born and raised in Manhattan there was pressure to dress to impress from a very early age. Now I dress for me."

real life: "I find myself in 'difficult' fashion situations on a weekly, sometimes daily basis, which is why the ability to transform is so much a part of my personal style. At least once a week an event will pop up that I hadn't anticipated—a cocktail party after work, a black-tie gala, or an important business dinner. Since the office is far from home and I can't go home to change I need to be able to take whatever I'm wearing and make it instantly appropriate for the occasion."

dianne vavra

VP of Public Relations, Dior Beauty

TRADE SECRETS

BLOUSES

TREAT BLOUSES IRREV-ERENTLY—MORE LIKE TANKS OR T-SHIRTS.

Blouses used to have a prim, fussy reputation. Now any kind of blouse you own is hip. Blouses will lift your wardrobe out of the T-shirt syndrome. Spice them up with heels and a shapely pencil skirt. Relax "good" silk blouses by layering them casually under V-necks and cardigans with jeans or khakis. Don't get hung up on size. Older silk blouses from decades past may be generously cut. That's fine; just remove any existing shoulder pads. The beauty of blouses is their fluid, drape-y look, so undo a few buttons at the neck and sleeves or let shirttails drift free. Retro details like big bows and peplums are bonuses.

Eve Fueur

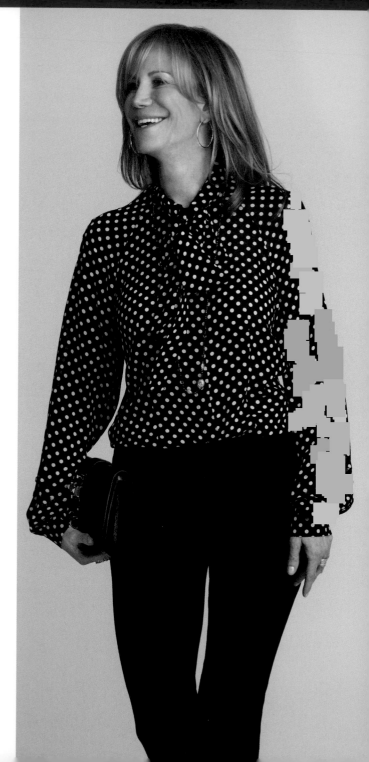

CARDIGANS

TIME FOR YOUR TWINSETS TO DIVORCE AND FOR YOU TO GET CREATIVE.
I hope you have plenty of cardigans because they're the acrobats of your closet, providing more tricks than any other basic. They do a great job providing arm coverage for sleeveless dresses but there's more in their repertoire than that.

- **A-shape them.** Start with the classic cardigan, the kind you see in twinsets (and please break them up ASAP simply because it's more youthful than a matched duo). Fasten only the top button and you get an A-line shape that defines your shoulders and arms but gently trapezes out to hide bra bulge and any muffin tops.

- **Blouson them.** Take the same cardigan and fasten only the last three buttons at the bottom instead. Then pull the sweater up so the hem sits at the top of your hip to create a subtle blouson shape. Push up the sleeves to ¾ length. You get definition and a lean line at the hip but the look provides ease and camouflage for a full bosom or flabby midriff.

- **Reverse them.** This is a great after work trick for dinner, cocktails, or a party. Switch your cardigan around back to front so the buttons go down your spine. Leave the bottom button or two open for ease over your hips. This gives any cardigan a subtle provocative look and is great over a slim pencil skirt or narrow cropped pants. Add a slim metallic belt (buckle at the front) to increase definition at the waist. For a slightly relaxed or sexier neckline, open two buttons at the nape. Don't worry, the sleeves and belt will keep all in place. This reversal trick works with V-neck cardigans, too, but the depth of the V will affect your button strategy.

- **Belt them.** Button only the middle buttons for shape when belting a cardigan over a dress. A pop-of-color cardigan belted over a neutral dress can add warmth, energy, and a youthful look. Wear cardigans loose over jeans, however—it's the time they really need to be open and free.

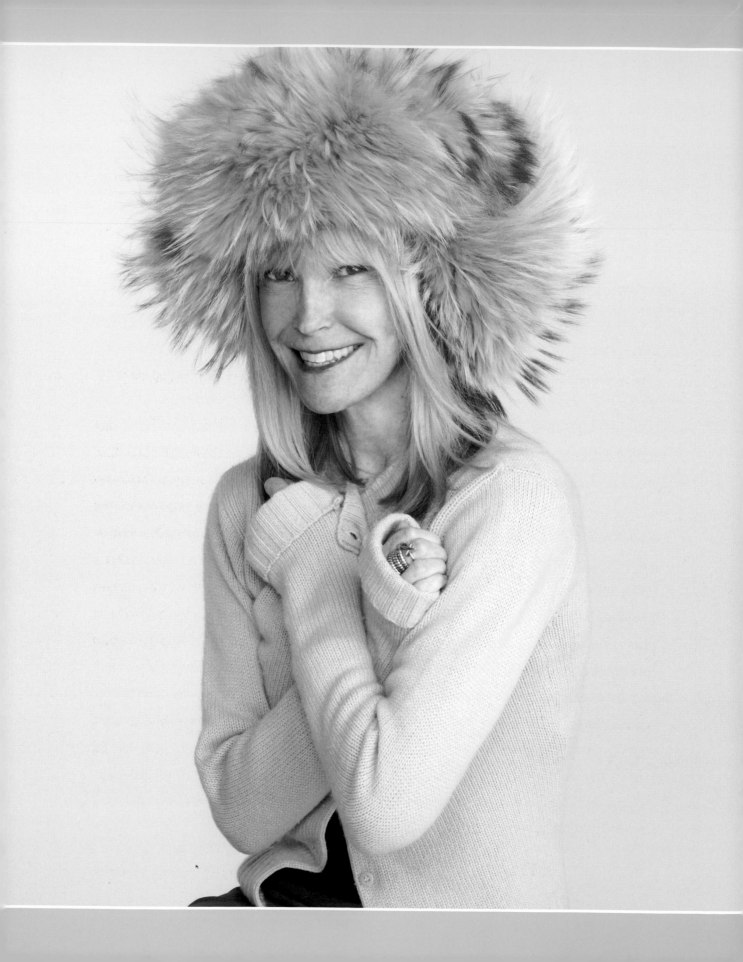

DRESSES

THEY'RE CLEARLY WORKHORSES NOW.

Use any tailored dress as a versatile base for all your jackets, cardigans, boots, and shoes of any height and shape. Get old dresses retailored to your current body. Any semi-fitted, curve-skimming sheaths and shifts with straps wide enough to cover your bra straps and a high neckline are the ones to focus on. Pull out dresses you might have once considered eveningwear only. Fabrics like brocade, velvet, taffeta, and metallic transition to day with nude pumps, a hobo or satchel, and low-key jewelry, hair, and makeup.

HATS

THOSE MEANT FOR OUTDOORS ARE KEEPERS.

• **Head warmers:** For warmth or inclement weather, five hat styles work for us: a fur trapper (real or faux) with ear flaps, a black beret, knit ribbed pull-on hats, slouchy knit beanies, and cowls that convert from neck warmer to hood. Start with black since a black hat with black gloves, a black bag, and black shoes sharpen the look of any coat you own. Go for other neutrals toned to your outerwear. Skip pastels, pompoms, anything print, or striped—forever.

• **Genuine sun protection:** Get serious about sun damage and skin cancer. Even if you wear a high-protection sun block, you need a brim that shades your face, neck, and ears. A cotton crusher (in any neutral), or a simple big-brimmed sunhat in woven straw or raffia are your two choices (helenkaminski.com and hat attack.com have the best). A baseball cap is not going to work for sun protection since it leaves your neck and ears exposed.

Really jam any hat on your head and do not perch it on top of your hair. Make this easier (and get more style points) by first pulling your hair into a low ponytail at the nape of your neck or sliding your hair flat behind your ears and skip the earrings.

Lois in her favorite Adrienne Landau trapper hat

JEANS

TRADE SECRETS

- **Classic jeans:** If yours are broken in, washed-out, classic straight-leg/five-pocket jeans like those by Levi's, Gap, J.Jill or J.Crew, wear them with attitude and a great belt. They're fantastic and sexy—and they, like us, get better with age.

- **Fashion jeans:** These are trendy jeans that mold to your tush and need frequent updates and editing to still look okay. Those currently in your closet may be straight, skinny, cropped, or bootcut, but keep it simple. Toss oldies with extras like studs, pockets, statement logos, extra-wide flares, or low rises. **The darker and more even the wash the dressier your fashion jeans are and the more easily they tone with your navy and black tops for a slim look.**

- **The right shoes/boots for jeans:** You need ankle cropped boots that won't create bulges or bulk beneath jeans legs. If you don't have them, get them. Choose the heel height that works with your jeans. Flat-cropped boots that hug the ankles slip beneath cropped or skinny jeans. Skinny jeans fitted all the way to the ankles and cropped jeans also look great with ballet flats, loafers, and flat sandals, or can be tucked into knee-high boots. Don't try tucking straight jeans or bootcuts into your knee-high boots. It's also time to give up the discomfort of wearing your knee-high boots under jeans. If you almost always wear bootcuts or relaxed straight-leg jeans you'll want a little extra jeans length puddling at the hem to compensate for width. Wear these with a short-cropped "bootie" with a walk-able chunky heel or wedge.

PANTS

YOU HAVE TWO CHOICES—CROP YOUR PANTS AT THE ANKLES OR WEAR HIGH HEELS. FRANKLY, I'D GO WITH OPTION #1 FOR EVERYDAY. Pant trends come and go but only two proportions matter: long and cropped. At this moment you probably have some of each in your closet but be ruthless in your editing—those that don't work need to go.

- **Ankle-cropped:** I hope you have these since they are comfortable, look fashionable with flats (but work with heels, too), provide a trim base for any top, and look modern as part of a pantsuit. Lots of women (editors, stylists, and even designers) use the term capris, cigarette pants, and cropped pants interchangeably. The fit and length are what matter, not the name. **Just above the anklebone is the right length for us**—not several inches above or covering the ankle to the top of the shoe. Even an inch in either direction makes a difference, so be fussy and have a tailor tweak any you own. The fit should be body skimming, not tight or molded to your skin. Get rid of wide cropped pants, especially those that hit your leg mid-calf or swing out in a flare. They make everyone look shorter and wider—like you're standing in a ditch. Honestly, they do.

- **Long:** If you prefer wearing longer pants with heels, stick to those with a straight, classy shape rather than an exaggerated wide-leg cut. Here's why: Wide-leg pants need extra length to compensate for the width; otherwise you look like a box. When pants get wider and longer, shoes need to go higher to compensate for the extra length. You can't win. Whenever you see an upswing in towering heels and platform wedges you can be sure long wide pants are not far behind. Let me burst your fashion bubble forever. Those long, slouchy full pants may look sexy swaggering down the runway on models but they do not hide fat or make you look six-feet tall. Wear your wide pants only if you're naturally tall and slim and have no problem with super-high heels because you'll need them to pull off the look. For shorter women, the combo of long full pants and high heels produces a weird walking-on-stilts illusion. The "leg" is all pant and shoe. Disaster!

RAINCOATS

A TRENCH IS FOREVER.

I bet you have at least one trench since they are truly timeless (and ageless). A classic knee-grazing trench in a tan/beige color and a water-resistant or waterproof fabric is the most useful coat you can own. If it has a removable lining, even better (yes, you do use the lining!). Throw on your trench, a black sweater, a skirt or cropped pants, black heels or flats, sunglasses, and you have an instant look. Whenever I have five minutes to pull myself together (and this happens a lot), this is what I wear. A trench looks just as right over a cocktail dress or jeans. To look chic, don't do the buckle. Just tie the belt in a knot and let the ends and buckle dangle. If you're wearing your trench open, knot the belt in the back or tuck the ends of the belt in your pockets. On truly rainy days, add a long scarf or cowl to flip up over your hair, waterproof boots, a cross-body bag (to leave your hands free for an umbrella), and you have instant style instead of a soggy mess.

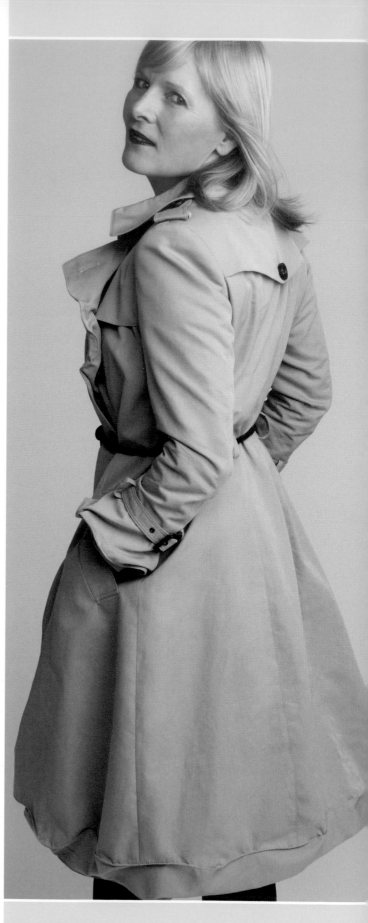

Annemarie Iverson in a Burberry "special edition" trench

Skirts

Classic knee-ish skirts like pencils and A-lines never die. Slightly fuller skirts with knife pleats, stitched down, inverted, or drop pleats can still work, but need strategy. Your keepers will be the right length: to the top, middle, or bottom of the knees or an inch or two above the knees, but no longer or shorter than that. Edit out tight minis and pencils that inch up your thighs when you sit and cross your legs.

Wearing a skirt means dealing with the break at the waist. Here's how:

- **Wear a matching flat-knit top or sweater over the skirt.** Emphasizing the vertical line makes skirts look slim and fashionable. You then have the option of defining the waist with a skinny belt over the sweater. An opaque shapewear bodysuit worn as a base layer can help smooth bulges and provides the security of a tucked-in piece without creating bulges.

- **Slim skirts can take a fitted or full jacket:** For example, pencil skirts easily balance the width of loose cropped jackets.

- **Full skirts need a fitted sweater or jacket:** When skirts are full at the bottom, the tops need to be more fitted.

Shirts

Any shirt looks better unbuttoned to a V just above your bra to show your collar-bones and elongate your neck. Our shirt collections are eclectic and may include classic Brooks Brothers button-downs, washed-out chambrays from college, fancy whites with French cuffs, and even ex-husband shirts. Whatever the case, never just put on your shirt—style it! Unbutton it to a V, gently tug the neckline to relax it, and then roll the sleeves casually

or push them up, leaving the cuffs flipped. Layer your shirts over tanks or slip them under V-necks and cardigans. Don't worry about a few wrinkles or the tails sticking out since a slightly rumpled effect is fine, especially with more casual looks.

SWEATERS

YOUR SLIM, FLAT-KNIT, HIP-LENGTH PULLOVERS AND CARDIGANS ARE THE MOST PRACTICAL ONES YOU OWN. Wear any long, slim sweater and pant/skirt duo in a matched or toned color and immediately you have a modern base for strong accessories. Add a tailored coat in a matching or toned color and you have an elegant, put-together look. Wear these sweaters belted over your bottom pieces for instant chic or with a matching flat-knit scarf for a new kind of "twinset."

What about all the chunky knits in your closet? Wear them on a home-alone night with a good movie and a fire or get rid of them!

TAILORED JACKETS

TOSS JACKETS ON LIKE CARDIGANS. We used to live for jackets. Back in the day, there was nothing like a blazer with shoulder pads to make us feel better about our hips and rear. But jackets have changed. New ones fit body-close and have stretch. Get your tailor nipping the shape and start treating jackets more like sweaters; don't be precious about them. Belt your most conservative ones to sex up the silhouette. Pair classic jackets with unexpected pieces to shake things up. You might wear a crisp navy blazer over a cashmere hoodie with slouchy gray cords. Try adding refined, ladylike jackets to sporty pieces for contrast.

TURTLE-NECKS

ONLY LEAN, STRETCHY TURTLES DO ANYTHING FOR YOU. Lots of women adore turtle-necks for their coverage of age-related issues and have collected them for years. Here's the hitch: a turtle really needs stretch and a sec-ond-skin fit from neck to hip to do you any good. I like solid black and neutral turtlenecks toned to whatever is on the bottom. I saw Ellen Barkin at a screening of her film *Another Happy Day* wearing a black super-fitted turtleneck sweater and lean black pants and wanted to run home and change my clothes to exactly the same thing.

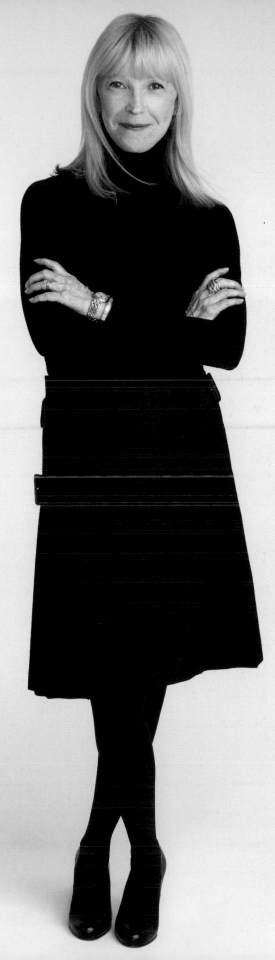

I'm Obsessed with . . .

Very few of us are at our so-called ideal weight. Even when the scale makes us smile we notice stuff has drooped and shifted. And guess what? Our bodies don't age symmetrically (just like faces!). One shoulder may be a little higher; one boob bigger or droopier; sun damage may show more on your cleavage and legs than your back or arms. Don't let any of this discourage you. Here's the bottom line when body meets fashion:

Style triumphs and learning to dress your body-of-the-minute well is the key to looking great in clothes old and new no matter what your age.

Still worried your aging body will jeopardize your newly de-aged wardrobe? Here's the solution: find a new "hot" zone; shift the focus somewhere else. These tips come with a flattery-back guarantee. If your issue is:

Big chest: Lots of women 40+ say weight gain and water retention show first in their chest and change the way clothes fit and look. Get over your fear of "big bras" and outsmart your body with a full-coverage minimizer or shaping bra. It will contain, center, and lift your boobs *without* adding extra cleavage or a rigid cardboard look under your clothes. Check out minimizers and full-coverage bras by Le Mystère, Wacoal, SPANX, and Chantelle. Then head for your wide V-necklines and wrap dresses when you're feeling top-heavy or puffy. But above all revel in your chest and let's remember being bosomy never bothered Elizabeth Taylor.

My Aging Body.

Disappearing waist: We all lose some body definition after 40 and nearly every woman complains about a flabbier middle. Bodysuits (in a leotard shape with a snap crotch) create the ultimate smoothest line under clothes. Wear them in place of tanks as "tuck-in" first layers under slim skirts, pants, and jeans to flatten and camouflage.

Flat derriere: Stick to dresses and skirts that skim over your rear or slide on butt-boosting shapewear pieces (SPANX Booty-Booster Short is like a bra for your derriere!) under your clothes. Check old knits and pants you wear a lot for a saggy bottom view and delete them if they do.

Fleshy un-toned arms: First of all, you notice this more than anyone else so don't give up entirely on baring your arms. To wear sleeveless more comfortably, fake your way to a slightly firmer look with gradual self-tanner (do your legs, neck, and face too for balance). Otherwise, make ¾ sleeves, lots of bracelets, and a flawless manicure (in the hottest new color) your new signature. By revealing the forearm you show only the slimmest, firmest part of your arm (implying the rest is just fine) while the jewelry and polish provides a diversion. Have your tailor shorten your long sleeve tees to ¾ ones—T-shirts, tops, dresses, jackets included. You can also simply push up the sleeves. Also, toning up your arms with weights— just enough to go bare and sleeveless—is a realistic goal since arms shape up faster than any other body zone.

Full, muscular calves: Toned calves seem marathon-runner powerful in a good way. You can balance the attention to your legs by showing off your arms. Wear straight-leg jeans, slim pants, and knee-high boots to give your legs a more uniform shape. Stay away from really high heels with skirts; the elevation causes leg muscles to tense, increasing the bulge of your calves.

My "new apple shape" with tummy: Changes in body-fat distribution as hormone levels shift, metabolism slows, and a fondness for cupcakes creeps in can result in belly bulge. So work on elongating your neck and legs, and wear straight shifts, A-lines, empire or raised waist dresses, and slim pants with long, layered tops or tunics. Put the emphasis at the neckline with a cowl, V-neck, or an eye-catching whopper of a necklace.

My new pear shape: Where did those thighs, hips, and derriere come from? Never mind, just make the most of your slim waist. This is actually a common shape for women over 40. So long as the difference between top and bottom doesn't get extreme you can work it. Wear more A-line dresses (fitted through the top and flared below) and A-line skirts instead of tapered pencils. Make belts your "new-again" favorite thing since you want to highlight that excellent waist. And choose relaxed jeans or khakis instead of tight jeans when you layer up.

Saggy chest: First thing to do is get a molded T-shirt bra. Constructed from light foam pre-formed into a firm permanent shape, these bras raise your boobs off your midriff and fill in volume on top for a youthful contour. They work best for the dual issue of size and sag. If your chest is small to medium, any smooth seamless microfiber underwire will do the trick—just add a V-neckline for a subtle, youthful sexiness. Let's consider mature, stylish French women; they're not obsessed with breasts being pushed up below their chins in an artificial way and neither should you. Since when is that a sign of style?!

Soft untoned hips and thighs: Easy. Psyche yourself firm with a pair of shapewear bike shorts from waist to thigh. The compression will immediately remind you of the tight and toned feeling you used to get from exercise and make all your clothes feel better. Just do it and don't complain about the compression—the tradeoff is worth it and easier than spinning or Zumba.

Spotty, veiny legs: Even five star legs may have broken capillaries, brown spots, or noticeable veins now. These are all normal characteristics of mature skin and sun damage. Don't let them stop you from wearing anything. Nude fishnets or a gradual self tanner can blur discolorations and provide a more even look while you play up your elongated legs in their nude pumps. If you self-tan, be sure to do your arms, face, neck, and backs of your hands too so that any exposed skin is the same color. You'll feel more comfortable going barelegged in skirts and dresses (and at the gym or pool, too).

The Top Mistakes Most Women Make With Their Old Clothes

During my thirties and early forties I explained every purchase to my guilty brain with, "I'll wear it forever!" Of course what survived are basic cashmere sweaters (those the moths didn't get), a few really good jackets and coats, a Burberry trench, Chanel bags, and my oldest jeans. They still look great decades later but I do miss other items I chucked way too easily. I miss my Sonia Rykiel knits from the '70s and '80s, my Lothar denims, and my Calvin Klein silk blouse and skirt duos from the '70s (very Faye Dunaway in *Network*). I search online auctions and consignment shops in vain for them every so often. Sometimes we keep hoarding or giving away the wrong things.

LET'S ALL STOP:

Thinking absolutely all classics are timeless. You probably bought straight skirts, crisp blazers, little black dresses, work suits, cashmere twinsets, and pleated menswear pants thinking you'd still wear them at age 90. Well even classics change. Now all of the above have a slimmer silhouette, improved fabrics, and updated details. Hold onto your pea coats, trenches, and riding jackets with nipped waists and see your tailor ASAP for the rest of it.

Keeping clothes for a lifestyle and body that's moved on. We dated, danced, partied, and had a blast in big fake jewels, sexy halters, sequins, and glitz. But here's a heads-up: Anything that now squeezes and blatantly shows too much flesh also reveals extra pounds, flab, and sag. Light reflecting surfaces always look bigger than they really are—great when it comes to jewelry, not so great when it comes to your derriere or chest.

Wearing long skirts. You don't need mid-calf length "midi" skirts, bohemian broomstick skirts, or bell-shaped ballroom skirts even if they're Ralph Lauren. Don't get romanced by the swirl or ability to cross your legs and forgo shapewear. The exception? A woman of extraordinary artsy bohemian style who has made long skirts her everyday signature. Tailor rehab can often produce knee-length chic skirts from long ones if the fit is straight and slim to start. This is often the case with buttery suedes and leathers.

Pairing over-the-knee boots with dresses. Thigh-high boots are a tricky call because they look okay or even great on trendy women with the right kind of body. But tall, slim knee-high boots are honestly just as effective for 99 percent of us. Wear your over-the-knee boots in black or neutrals toned to dark opaque tights or sweater-dresses. Also try them with skinny jeans and layers.

Letting the size on the label go to your head. Let's start by agreeing size is truly meaningless. A closet of multiple sizes doesn't mean "eating disorder alert!" You can wear a size 4 at Ann Taylor, an 8 at J.Crew, and a 6 in Michael Kors. In recognition of our weight and diet obsession, the smart fashion biz keeps rolling out smaller sizing to appease our vanity. So we have XXS, XS, 00, 0, and 2. There is absolutely no standard designer to designer, brand to brand. Don't pay attention to size. Remove the size tab after you buy!

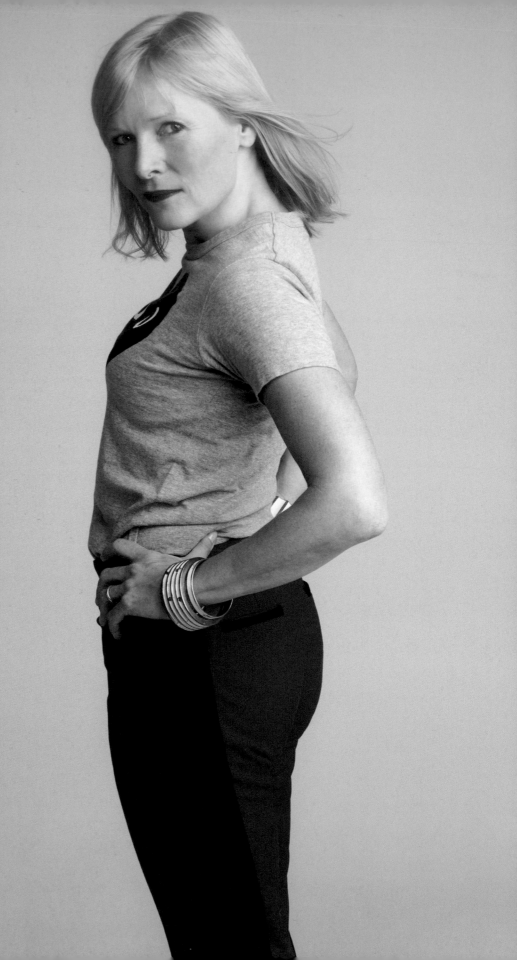

a n n e m a r i e

annemarie on:

style: "My look is tailored and elegant but also personal and relaxed. I tend to set a 'look' for the season—say five to ten daytime outfits that work for me for a few months. This saves me time in the morning without compromising the feeling that I look well-dressed and original. This season I'm into red and trying to wear pants a lot more. I made two or three investment purchases and these items are the center of my look."

age and fashion: "I think wearing things the way they come down the runway or as they are on the pages of a fashion magazine or blog is boring and aging. I love mixing things up! Although I could wear junior-sized clothing and slinky dresses or skimpy shorts I don't feel it's appropriate to do so. I'm a mom, a professional, and a wife, and even in my downtime want to dress appropriately."

annemarie iverson

Senior VP Creative Brand Development, Estée Lauder Companies; former editor-in-chief of *Seventeen* and *YM* and beauty and fashion news director of *Harper's Bazaar*

CHAPTER TWO

MONEY CHANGES EVERY-THING

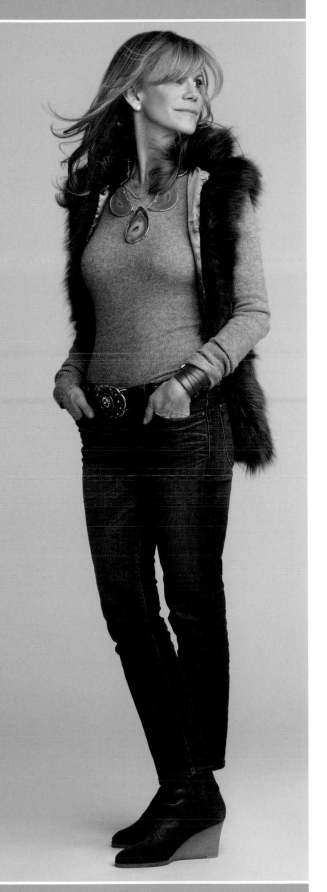

But style and taste don't have a price tag.

We all want to spend less but dress better. Every single woman 40+ I know cross-shops lower down the fashion chain than ever before. Sure, we're still interested in luxury brands but not quite as infatuated. Fast fashion is our new flirtation. Not long ago we stalked department store sales for markdowns or shopped Loehmann's and Filene's Basement for bargains. Nabbing designer clothes—any designer—at an incredible discount was the ultimate coup. Now we have a broader strategy for shopping and a new interest in labels and stores with a hip, lower-priced sensibility. We comparison shop online and get fashion alerts for items we want on sale. We mix Zara and J.Crew with our own "vintage" wardrobe pieces. We add a few basics from H&M, Target, or Gap and splurge once in a while and we're actually pretty happy . . . and well dressed. But when it comes to big spenders, honey we broke the mold.

Eve Feuer

Here's the
real backstory

Fashion works for us, not the other way around. It's ironic. Here we are, the generation of women that made big-name designers desirable, available, and affordable for all (if you count pantyhose, sunglasses, and perfume). We were loyal and kept buying even while prices escalated. Now we've decided enough is enough. We're making new choices. Fashion is now driven mostly by youth and celebrities, designers who are essentially rock stars, and low-cost super-stores. It's a fast, competitive, and sometimes annoying industry but our huge demo of women 40+ still has the influence to make or break brands and trends. Let's not forget:

- **We invented the bohemian thing.** Our minis, tie-dyed tees, embroidered tunics, midi skirts, and frayed bells created a new fashion niche. Vintage jeans? Hippie chic? We lived it.

- **We inspired designers to think small. If we couldn't buy the jacket we bought the bag, the scarf, the shoes, or the belt.** We built the small luxury-goods empire dollar by dollar and lots of us have the stuff to prove it.

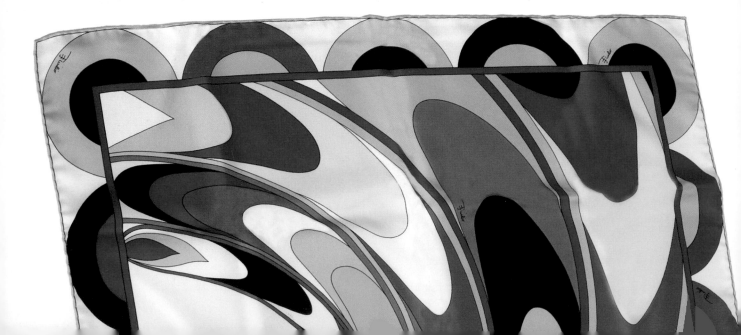

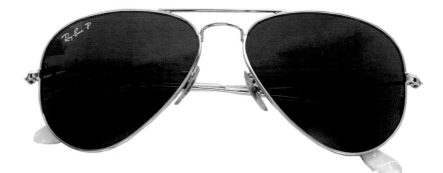

- **We developed the minimalist neutral idea.** We toned it down by the 1990s. We encouraged Donna and Calvin to give us subtle colors like taupe and gray, and Ralph to keep us in "good taste."

- **We made Lycra and spandex the real fashion success story of the century.** We roused the lingerie industry to give us seamless microfiber bras, thongs, and shapewear that didn't look like our mothers' girdles.

- **We bought tons of chic sweats, leggings, and yoga clothes.** They let us cheat guilt-free on workouts and diets and made us feel healthier just dressing like gym bunnies.

- **Then we made an executive decision. We decided comfort and convenience were never going to be negotiable again.** We inspired a shoe revolution and ballet flats, driving shoes, and comfort pumps (with padded, sneaker-like insoles) became the new basics.

- **Now fast forward to our favorite new formula: big sunglasses, cropped capris, and flats.** It was love at first try-on. Our new greeting isn't about a label or impressing one another. It's simply "You look great!"

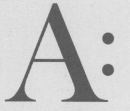

Question & Answer

Q: Do you secretly believe low-cost clothes make you look cheap?

A: You need to know where to draw the line.

The idea of looking cheap really scares us. We know money can't guarantee taste or style but it can often buy quality. We never want to look cheesy and that's where fast fashion goes haywire. The prices, merchandise, quality, and fit vary wildly so you need to find your comfort level. How low you go is up to you. The truth is there are plenty of affordable and moderately priced clothes with loads of style, but there are even more low-cost options without a trace of it. Learning to weed out the good stuff is the goal. Here are the facts of low-cost fashion life after 40.

What spending less can do for you now

It can save you from fashion debt, for starters. It can also get you out of a style rut and shake up clothes that feel dull or dated. How many more reasons do you need? We all overspend and buy clothes we can't afford. Our disposable income may have taken a hit, and our tastes, needs, and bodies may have changed but we still love looking good.

All the women photographed for *The Wardrobe Wakeup* either cross-shop the high/low spectrum, do vintage, or shop their closet more and stores less. For this book, I also interviewed hundreds of other women in their forties, fifties, and beyond who claim an allergy to low-cost clothes. I sense a growing fear that anything less than designer clothes can cross the border into dowdy/young/cheesy/frumpy land, especially after 50. Here's how to get past the label and make affordable fashion a bigger part of your life.

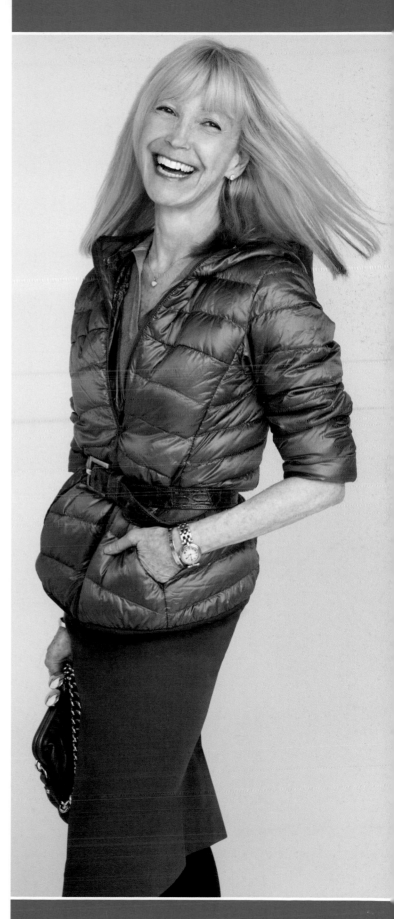

Lois wears a Uniqlo quilted jacket and Barneys skirt: mix of high and low

It's the magic mix of color, proportions, accessories, and your body that make fashion work for you—not the name on the label.

Me too! Same thing! I used to like—make that *love*—wearing totally recognizable labels and logos. As a young fashion editor having the newest "whatever" designer/item of the minute made me feel successful and confident. Now I prefer unidentifiable items whatever they cost. In fact, the more unidentifiable the better. I usually cut all inside labels out of my clothes to make them more me (a quirk, but true). After decades of snobby designer addictions I've become a cheap chic convert. Some of it has to do with my major lifestyle/work switch but I'm also enjoying dressing purely for me, not my job, my colleagues, or my industry.

It's been freeing. If you're raking in a nice salary and can afford $1,995 for a Donna Karan dress or $695 for Jil Sander pants and that's fine for you, don't let me get in your way. Some items are worth the splurge for the fit, versatility, look, and pure pleasure of wearing—although if you can get them for less why not? Let me point out some low-cost items are perfect too for their fit, versatility, and look and also deliver a totally pleasurable style experience. The idea is to integrate these items into your existing wardrobe, not to start over from scratch. Even die-hard fashionistas with a history of buying and wearing the crème de la crème of clothes can learn to love malls and mass market.

LOIS' HOTSHOT FASHION EDITOR

Class #2

10 Spend Less, Dress Better Tricks to Know

1. Print dresses are always a smart, low-cost buy.

Ever since Diane von Furstenberg and Pucci hooked us on print dresses back in the '70s we've known they were a fast, flattering, feminine solution for body and style. Now print dresses are all over the moderately priced market. We love the way prints camouflage jiggles and bulges and manufacturers love the way they hide inexpensive fabrics and imperfect construction—so it's a win-win. Tailored sheaths and crisp shifts look sophisticated in neutral abstract or graphic prints and trendy in bolder colors and splashy florals. Just watch the length and skip minis. The jerseys, especially those with sleeves, are usually lowest in terms of cost and are ideal for summer, warm climates, and travel since they're comfortable, crease-free, and require no extra layers for coverage. If you've never really worn print dresses before, start with those in your favorite neutrals to easily integrate them into your wardrobe. I'm a huge fan of the very affordable jersey print dresses by Ali Ro, JB by Julie Brown, and Donna Morgan.

Make swirly abstracts, florals, and animal prints that keep the eye moving your first choice since the free-flow disguises awkward pattern breaks at the seams, hem, and neckline.

2. Anchor a lower-cost look with an expensive item.

Few women over forty can wear cheap clothes head to toe and look great. You always need the push of one posh item or accessory to lift the look. Mix your more economical finds with splurges from your past, vintage accessories, or a new consignment shop find.

> The expensive "lift" item can be anything—a belt, shoes, a cashmere sweater, silk blouse, or a statement necklace—but you do need it.

Frankly, those cheapo get-this-look simulations with super low-cost clothes work only in magazine photos or on very young women. Here's how cheap does work: You might wear a black jersey dress from Target with your own vintage belt, $10 "silver" hoops from the local flea market, and pricey Stella McCartney metallic gladiator sandals snagged on sale. Or you might wear new black pants from Gap with a black shirt from Lands' End and a Prada belt.

3. Count on draping, shirring, and ruching, too.

Dresses, tops, and skirts that are ruched, shirred, or draped also disguise body flaws, budget fabrics, and low-cost workmanship. The mini folds used in ruching or shirring (same thing) blur bulges but keep body contours visible so you still have a sense of shape. The extra texture created by the gathers camouflages inexpensive or lightweight fabrics and provides a stylish detail. Draping fabric in more generous swaths here and there—usually across the stomach, hips, or at the neckline, works the same way. You'll see this use of fabric at every price point from fast fashion to couture.

Simple shapes and solid colors show off ruching and draping details best since the folds are visible, but wearing prints plus ruching or draping doubles your camouflage benefits.

Valerie Lynn wears a low-cost, ruched leopard dress with luxury brand boots

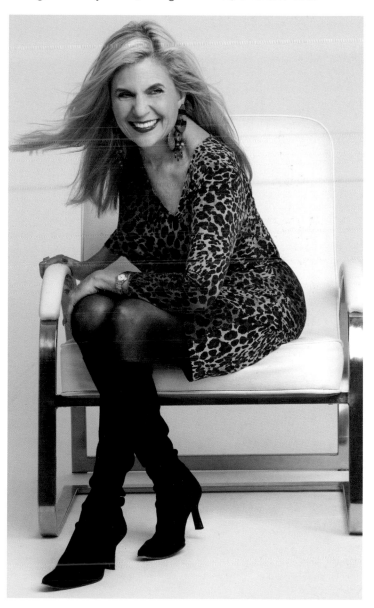

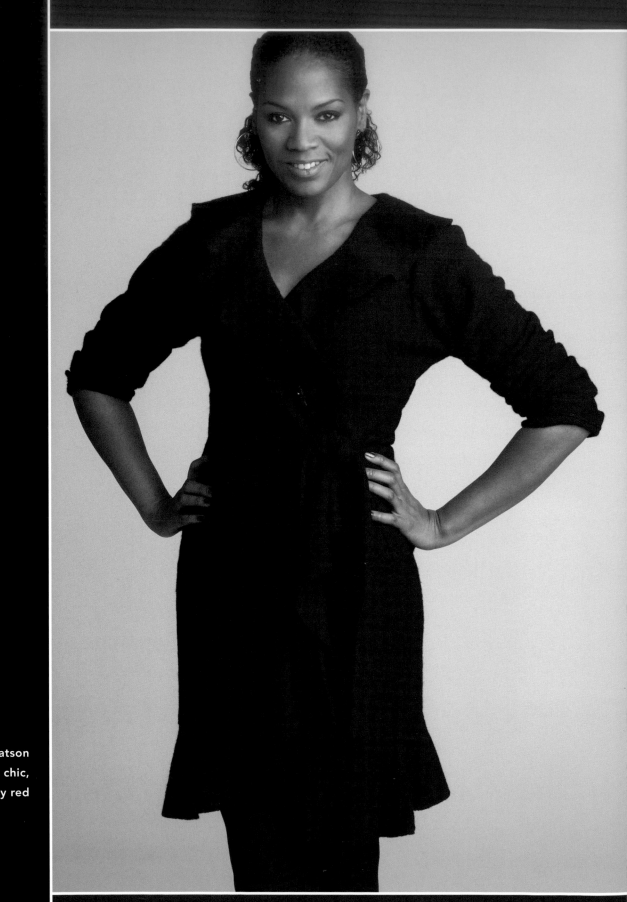

Cynde Watson
glows in chic,
classy red

4. Keep them guessing with gray, black, brown–or red!

To navigate the world of low-cost fashion but look like you're shopping high-end stores, you have to put on blinders. Be prepared to reject a lot of trendy, muddy colors, pastels, and blaring brights. Faking an upscale look means sticking to pared-down basics in clean shapes, a body-skimming fit, and the neutral colors that always look satisfyingly rich. Black, gray, navy, taupe, and brown may not be the most exciting colors but they always look classy. **If you absolutely crave color, buy classic red. It always looks in style and brightens mature skin like a dose of blusher.**

5. Get your white tees and camis at the drugstore.

There's honestly no reason to spend more since white cotton T-shirts, tanks, and camisoles stain and turn yellow or dingy gray no matter what you do. Buying inexpensive versions means no guilt when you toss them or use them to polish your shoes. Hanes plain ribbed cotton white tanks in a men's size small make amazing layering pieces. I've been wearing variations of these since the '80s.

6. Get into the fast fashion mood.

Fast fashion stores are where you see trends first, thanks to efficient teams that translate runway looks almost overnight. Stay fluid in attitude when navigating these fashion epicenters because they change quickly. Items we once considered super trendy, like platform shoes, python bags, and cropped leather jackets have become "new classics." Things we considered stuffy, like blouses, floral dresses, and frame bags, have become cool and trendy again. For those of us who like to explore trends in a safe way, one strategy works best: A low-cost classic in a trendy color, texture, or print can turn your closet around, but then so can a trendy item in a classic color.

7. Wear shapewear as a liner to improve fit.

When designers and manufacturers cut costs, linings are the first to go. These silky inner "skins" used to mean quality but now even pricier clothes scrimp on them. Linings do help tailored skirts, dresses, and pants keep their shape, but wearing control garments under inexpensive unlined items provides the same benefits. You don't need maximum strength shapewear—any silky, light compression piece will help clothes skim over stress points. Shapewear works as a buffer between unlined items and your skin. It prevents sticking and pulling so clothes won't crease, pull, or ride up as you bend and move.

Buy a bike short shaper in nude and black and one full shaper slip in black to improve the fit of tailored clothes and give lightweight items a firm, opaque base.

8. Satisfy trendy cravings with one "wow" item a season.

One trendy item can satisfy this urge without blowing your fashion strategy. It's like eating one fabulous cookie instead of completely falling off your diet. Just wear it for a season and get over it already.

Choose one small new statement piece to add to your usual clothes for an unexpected twist and pure fun.

FYI, this is also how stylists and editors punch up predictable or boring clothes and basics for editorial features in magazines. A leather tunic dress to wear over jeans or printed capris could add just enough "new" to keep you going.

9. Get your designer fix from consignment and eBay.

The leftovers from someone else's closet can provide the rush you used to get spending on new clothes minus the guilt. Think about it. You can get pricey fabrics and quality buying vintage for the same money you spend at mall-based chain stores. These clothes often have the kinds of details that are hard to find anymore, like seams bound with satin tape to prevent fraying, real silk linings on coats and jackets, skirts and dresses with hand-sewn deep hems and bound buttonholes. Start hunting now—before the twenty- or thirty-somethings get there. Here are some things I always look for that work for everyone:

Tailored, ladylike dresses and designer sheaths in bright colors: The fabrics and workmanship are perfect.

Leather pencil skirts: Remember waistbands can be narrowed or removed, mid-calf lengths shortened to knee-ish.

Jane Larkworthy

Beautiful white or ivory silk designer shirts: Go for silks that are fluid, opaque, and have some heft to the fabric (not lingerie weight). Check underarms for stains!

Capes and fur-trimmed ponchos: No kidding, a knee-length cloak is easy to throw over layers and looks great with pants, jeans, or skirts.

Bold faux jewelry: Cuffs, chain-link bracelets, chunky necklaces, pendants, and charms

Tailored coats with or without fur trim and designer trenches: The details and fabrics are luxurious.

Interesting belts from Hermès to vintage alligator ones from the '50s: To personalize any bargain dress and give jackets a new waist

10. Go up a size to improve fit.

Sometimes, in an effort to cut costs, manufacturers will pare down the amount of fabric used in lower cost clothing to the bare minimum. (Actually, they sometimes do this in expensive clothes, too!) This can leave the fit in your usual size feeling snug or skimpy. Relax the fit and get a more luxurious look by going for the next size. The fabric will have just enough room to drape and move on the body without stressing the small seam allowances.

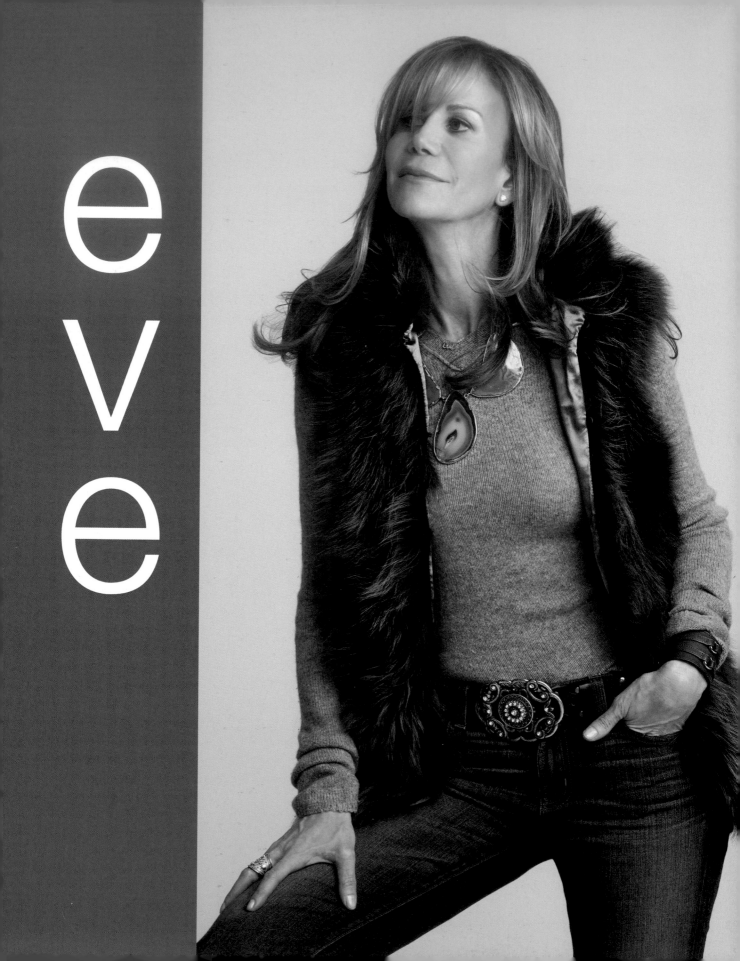

eve on:

age and fashion: "I am more comfortable with
my body now than when I was much younger and work out regularly to stay in shape. Because I don't feel my best wearing overtly
body conscious clothes, I'll pair a tight top with a loose pant or
vice versa. I'll use belts to create more definition when wearing a
dress or cardigan. I choose jeans with a higher rise to avoid a
"muffin top" and wear SPANX with dresses just to keep everything
smooth. I do think there is age-appropriate clothing and don't like
seeing moms dressing exactly the same as their daughters. No more
minis for me and I won't buy a dress if I can't wear a proper bra.
I won't buy shoes that are not comfortable anymore."

shopping: "I am definitely buying less because I tend
to repeat the same purchases with only a slight difference. I mix
brands and labels but know exactly who has what I love. For example, Zara always has perfect blouses. I can rely on Tory Burch and
J.Crew for great tweed jackets, J Brand for ideal jeans, Michael
Stars for my favorite V-neck T-shirts, Target for the best tanks,
and Inhabit for the best sweaters."

eve feuer

Celebrity stylist and wardobe consultant

TRADE SECRETS

LEARN FROM THE EXPERTS.

ONE OF THE WAYS TO GET MORE OUT OF DESIGNER CLOTHES WITHOUT ACTUALLY WEARING THEM IS TO STUDY HOW YOUR FAVORITE DESIGNERS COMBINE ELEMENTS, LAYER, AND USE DETAILS.

If you love fashion, nothing beats reading online or in magazines about the hottest trends of the season. Checking out designer runway shows on style.com is the closest most women get to buying couture or collection clothes. Watch and learn and then do your own interpretations at J.Crew, Zara, and Ann Taylor.

RENT A DRESS OR BAG.

YOU ESSENTIALLY RENT THE ITEMS YOU WANT AND PAY A MONTHLY FEE. THE TWO BEST ARE:

Renttherunway.com: Perfect dresses for weddings, parties, and events. Designers include Vera Wang, Alberta Ferretti, Badgley Mischka, Moschino, and Carmen Marc Valvo.

Bagborroworsteal.com: Rent a designer bag or jewelry by the week or month. Return via UPS or buy it when you're done. There's Louis Vuitton, Gucci, Prada, and more.

Lower your expectations.

WE WANT THAT $80 PENCIL SKIRT TO FIT AND FEEL LIKE ONE THAT COSTS $450. BUT IN THE END WE KNOW IT WON'T. You get more sizzle out of fashion from mixing high and low—one feeds off the other. Wear that new low-cost pencil skirt with your vintage designer jacket and you elevate the skirt and give the jacket a hipper, trendier attitude.

Sell what you don't wear.

BEFORE YOU BUY AN-OTHER THING, GET RID OF THE EXCESS. Selling old loves is a smart move, though donating your rejects to charity rates a tax deduction—just ask for and keep a receipt to file with your return. If you choose to sell via the consignment route, get a written contract that says what percentage of the sale price you get. Set a practical time limit since you want to be able to retrieve your stuff and donate it (if it doesn't sell) to still get that tax benefit. Selling on eBay is another option. Check the site first so you get a feel for the kind of photo and description that appeal to buyers. Pay attention to the positive feedback certain sellers get for items similar to the ones you want to sell.

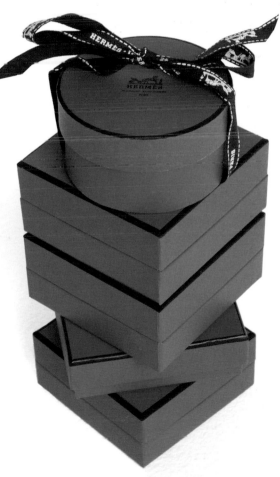

GET INTO DISCOUNT AND BONUS SITES.

FREE SHIPPING AND RE-TURNS AND ALERTS ARE POWERFUL LURES. Can't re-sist an extra 30 percent off alert in your inbox? During Cyber Monday last year I scored items I'd been on the fence about. Don't get trapped by the "take an additional 20 percent off" strategy some stores use on sale items. The second discount is on the reduced price, not the original price. You don't add the two together for a stunning total discount. Read the fine print and ask in store about any extra savings opportunities! Don't assume the price on the tag in any store is the final price.

Valerie Monroe in jeans, white tank, and pricey shoes from a Paris boutique

LOSE THE ATTITUDE.

FASHION SNOB-ISM IS FOR SUPERFICIAL WOMEN WITHOUT SUBSTANCE. THAT'S NOT US. Any woman with twenty or thirty years of retail experience in the shopping trenches knows how fickle fashion is and how today's trend is tomorrow's trash. Think about it—you know how we love to rate Red Carpet looks at the Oscars? Does our opinion depend on whether a dress is Lanvin or Versace? It's more like "she looked great" versus "she looked terrible." Remember Sharon Stone's Gap turtleneck (with a Valentino skirt) in 1996?!

TRY NEW ONLINE SOURCES.

YOU'LL FIND FRESH FASHION SITES AND STORES OPEN UP YOUR OPTIONS. You just might discover distinctive items for less money than you planned on spending. Shops that attract teens also have great deals, but watch out for skirt/dress lengths, waistbands and rises, and low necklines. At the mall or online stop in at: C. Wonder, American Apparel, and Madewell for unexpected finds. Online try: shopbop.com, revolveclothing.com, mytheresa.com, madisonplus.com (for sizes 14 to 28), and the outnet.com.

GIVE IT 24 TO 48 HOURS.

NO MATTER WHAT IT IS, THINK ABOUT IT. LAST ONE? CHECK THE RETURN POLICY. Demonstrate the self-confidence and discipline that comes only with age and wisdom. Put things on "hold" or in a virtual shopping bag instead of rushing to buy. Give it a weekend. If the initial passion is over by Monday it was a fling and not worth the involvement. If it's gone you were never meant to have it (as my mother always said and now I do, too).

TRADE SECRETS

I'm Obsessed with . . .

Some women, particularly those who have a history of buying and wearing expensive clothes, look down their noses at fast fashion. Here are some ways to deal. If you're worried about looking:

Classy not cheap. Worried someone will out you as a bargain hunter? Puh-leeeze we're all doing it. Stock up on feminine tops, like silky blouses, classic fitted V-necks, and cardigans in neutral colors, perfect button-front shirts, tailored dresses, ballet flats, trenches, and slim ankle cropped pants.

Professional even at bargain prices. Inexpensive work clothes are trickiest for grown-up women in senior management level positions who need to look somewhat corporate. I like consignment shops if you really want a quality look for less here. Otherwise stick to expensive-looking neutrals colors that make it hard to pin down a price. Since jackets and pants require more meticulous attention to fit, select dresses and skirts as a first choice. Always add strong jewelry, a good leather bag and shoes, and everyone will assume you were a CEO in your previous life.

Youthful not ridiculous. Low-cost shopping is not about commitment, so you can take a few chances here. Look for newsy prints, upbeat colors, and the kind of shoes people notice. Add simple, playful touches one at a time. Keep the shapes classy, pump up the color, and update the fabric and details—items like a jersey pencil in rose pink, a black and white striped blazer, and red suede platform wedges should give you the idea.

Looking Well Dressed.

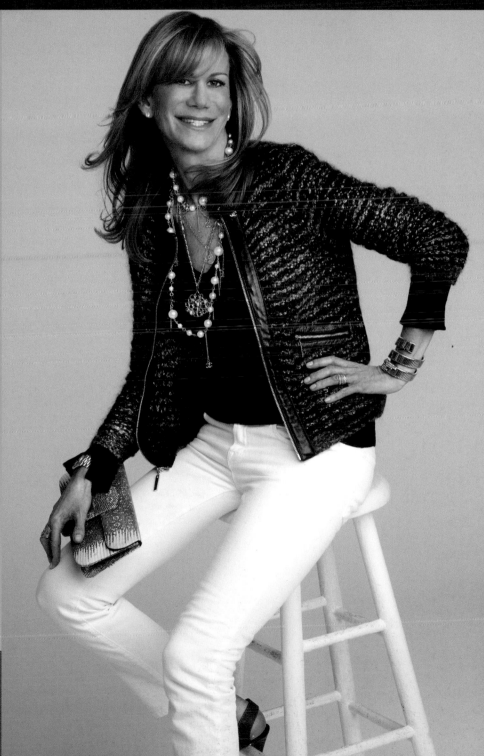

Eve Feuer in white jeans and Chanel jacket: mix of high and low

The Top Money-Saving Mistakes Women Make

Sometimes we go off track. It's fine. Think about how many eye shadows, lipsticks, and face creams you've bought that have been duds and you'll feel a whole lot better.

LET'S ALL STOP:

Buying "pretty" low-cost bras. You can't scrimp on bras after 40 if you have sag and size issues. Lacy, colorful, and decorative is gorgeous but it's not going to work without some serious support and that doesn't mean just an underwire. You want a bra that is smooth, seamless, lifts, supports, and doesn't make you bulge at the sides or back. Expensive bras will make any inexpensive top or dress look better.

Thinking flats are flats. Not all flats are created equal. It's easy to find chic, inexpensive ballet flats. Serious work flats require a touch more structure, a slightly thicker sole, a tapered toe, good quality leather, and no toe cleavage. This still leaves room for style: a jeweled ornament, cap toe, bow, quilting, or patent leather can all work. Sometimes they're also called skimmers—just to confuse you.

Not examining clothes inside and out: Do your due diligence when shopping. Look at the seams and stitching. Skip anything with irregular stitching, loose threads, puckered or unraveling seams, or pockets that are purely decorative as a design doo-dad. Be sure zippers slide easily and that the teeth lock at the bottom of jackets without a struggle. Test fabrics for crease resistance. Crunch and twist them in your hands, hold for a few seconds then release to see how quickly and easily the creases fall out.

Expecting teen-targeted clothes to work on our grown-up bodies. Some brands and stores really do not see us as their ideal customer. The fit model for some companies is a teen or twenty-something-year-old. So don't expect jackets with a defined waist to sit at your real waist and be the right length, or skirts to not be minis.

Turning up your nose at fast fashion. Stand in line at H&M and Target, where you can snag super-cheap finds from guest collaborators like Stella McCartney, Donatella Versace, Jason Wu, Missoni, Marni, Thakoon, and Rodarte to mix with your discounted high-end purchases. You're in for a surprise.

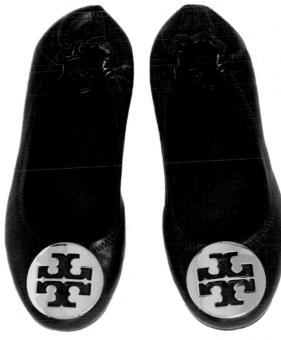

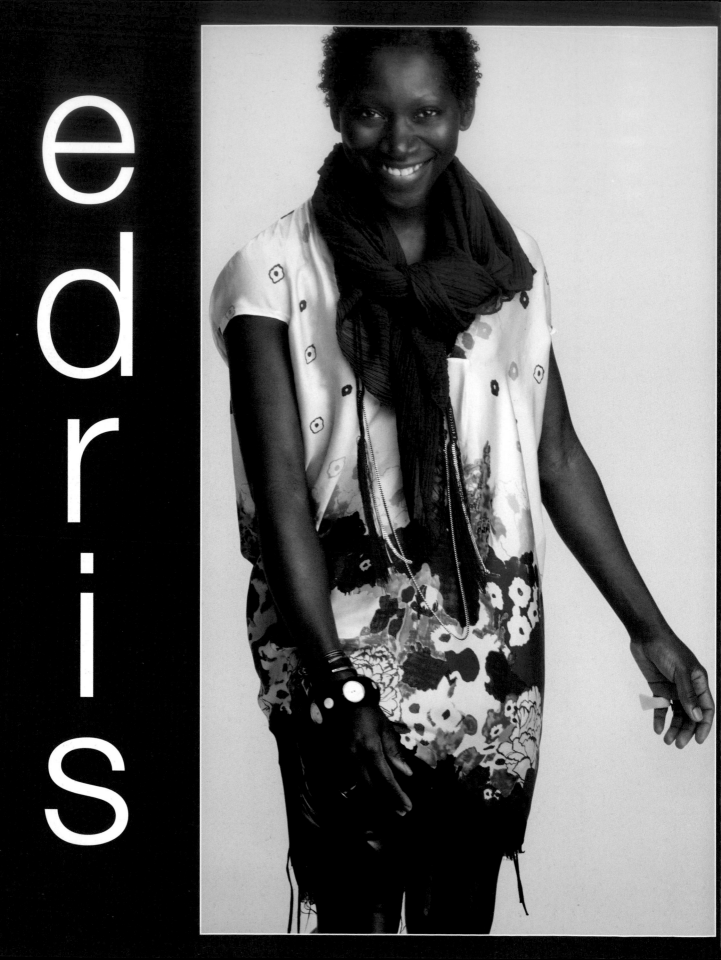

edris

edris on:

wardrobe: "If you love fashion as I do you hold no bias. My closet is a vault. I tend to hold on to quality pieces and have clothes from all designers but now I seek out young emerging designers like Ana Kata, a Nigerian designer I am mentoring. Most of my clothes are separates so I can mix and match them easily and add my daily dose of statement accessories—the necklaces, rings, scarves, and bags that are a big part of my look. I love accessories that wow me, especially original, eccentric one-of-a-kind pieces from artisans. Lately I've been picking up finds in Sydney, Australia from new designers. I collect American Indian jewelry, Art Deco pieces, and handcrafted items, so I'm always looking."

current obsession: "My purple Issey Miyake scarf is something I wear all the time, every day, with absolutely everything. A young Japanese woman told me historically only the highest monks wore purple. Why not have that positive energy around me? In general I love Issey Miyake—the clothes are fun, versatile, and have an architectural element."

edris nicholls

Owner Edris Salon, NYC, and Altelier Director at Shu Uemura

Things that always look great

Certain inexpensive items have eye, heart, and brain appeal. You'll find them everywhere, at every price, every year, but stick to the cheapies and snap them up as you go. You'll wear them to death and wish you'd bought a backup. Next time you will.

BLACK MATTE JERSEY DRESS: Throw it on over black leggings, tights, or bare legs. Look for any of these details: a defined waist or raised empire waist, draping or wrapping, a flattering V- or ballet-neck, and elbow length or ¾ sleeves.

CARDIGANS: Snap up classic flat-knits with round and V-necks; embellished styles with embroidery, beads, sequins, or decorative jewel trims; distinctive colors and animal prints; long, slim boyfriend styles to belt over dresses and skirts. You'll never have too many.

CASHMERE AND BLENDS: Since the price of cashmere just keeps going up, look for affordable, lightweight cashmere/cotton, or cashmere/silk blends. Even a small percentage brings a luxurious difference to a blended fabric. Look for flat-knit cardigans and pullovers to tone with your pants, skirts, and dresses—whatever your main base colors.

. . . even when they're dirt cheap.

CASUAL PANTS: They can be cargos, slim khakis, or stretchy cords but aim for a slim-fitted look through the waist, stomach, and hip, even if the leg is slouchier. You don't want any pants that are stiff, wide, or boxy. Some have a washed, broken in look, others are pressed and polished enough to sub for dress pants. Solid gray, beige, olive, black, or khaki will work best. They look great with ballet flats, loafers, driving moccasins, flip-flops, or sneakers. Roll the bottoms and add your most glam heels and a jacket to take them out to dinner or to the office.

CLUTCH BAGS: Soft leather pouches with a frame top are smarter for day than more structured styles since they adjust to fill. For evening look for fakery—beads, sequins, crystals. Embellished clutches are easy to hold in your hand or tuck under your arm.

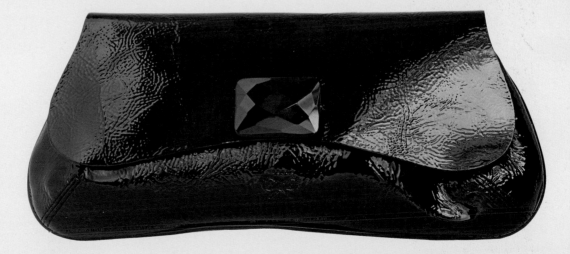

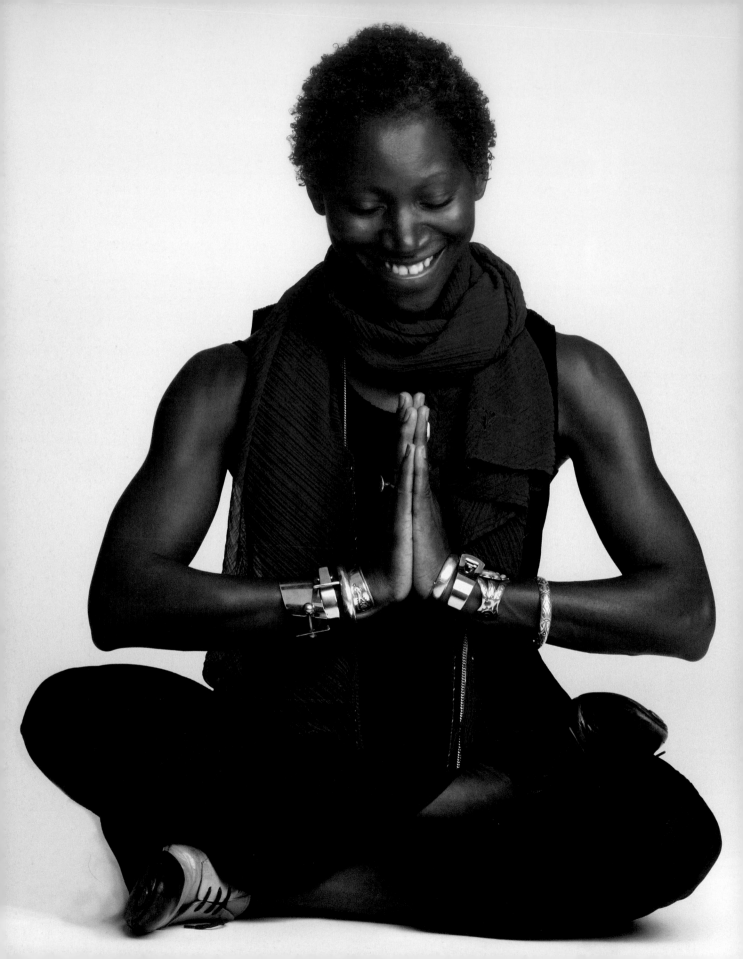

DRESSY HEELS: Sales are the best for gold, silver, jewel-embellished, or silk glitzy shoes. Splurge on practical black or nude pumps for work but never pay full price for party pumps!

GLAM EARRINGS: Look for lightweight state-ment earrings that won't stretch your piercings or lobes further—or the new clip on drops that are stress-free. Pick up inexpensive ethnic jewelry from India, Africa, and Mexico, too—gorgeous!

FLAT GOLD SANDALS: Thongs, gladiators, and strappy sandals in metallic leather and snakeskin are always in style and always a smart buy. What if you're more of a silver person? Snap those up, too. Gold and silver flats transform any base of black; give camel, brown, or white a jet-set gleam; and lift navy and gray out of the doldrums.

LONG SUPPLE SCARVES: These are the equivalent of necklaces, bringing color, light, and attitude to your face. Grab lightweight silky, rayon, modal, cotton, and wool blends in flattering colors and prints to drape at the neck. They are truly quick year-round look-changers.

SPARKLY FLATS: Ballet flats with jewels, crystals, or bedazzled with glitter give slim pants and jeans the feeling of dressy without having to wear heels.

SUNNIES: Oversized black sunglasses and aviators always look great and inexpensive versions make keeping backup pairs everywhere easy. Want to prevent crow's feet and squint lines or minimize UV damage to the eye area? This is one of the best ways—just be sure the lenses say "UV protection."

Edris Nicholls in black pants and top lifted by purple Issey Miyake scarf and Vivienne Westwood intentionally mismatched lace-ups

Lois' *Amazing* STYLE-FOR-LESS
Shopping Guide

American Apparel (americanapparel.com)

Don't let the super-young customers deter you. They have great basics in every color, including **T-shirts, cardigans, cotton sweaters, and clingy stretch cotton turtlenecks**. When you need a cheap layering piece in any neutral, head here. I bought a black synthetic knit beanie for $20 that looks every bit as great as my $500 cashmere one.

Ann Taylor (anntaylor.com)

Love the polished aesthetic and feminine styling that makes dressing for work or job-hunting after 40 affordable and stress-free. If you like **well-cut jackets and pants, beautiful blouses and dresses that look professional** but can't splurge on Piazza Sempione or Armani Collezioni, try Ann.

Banana Republic (bananarepublic.com)

For conservative updated suits, jackets with nipped waists, and an easy "fit" system for identifying the perfect pants, this brand is a good source. **The Logan slim fit ankle pants are ideal for petites** and the leather bags are luxurious looking, well priced, and get better with age.

Chico's (chicos.com)

If it's good enough for fashion icon Diane Keaton (who did a stint in their ads) it's okay for me. The overall vibe is global with lots of prints and ethnic-inspired jewelry, but I like the **soft stretch shirts and microfiber tanks, lightweight travel coats, and jackets perfect for a cruise or road trip.**

Gap (gap.com)

The **classic favorite tee** in crew and V neck styles are can't-miss basics, but check out the revolving stacks of boatnecks and blousons and slouchy draped tops. The GapFit workout clothes are great and the huge range of Gap 1969 Premium jeans in sizes 00 to 20 include classic and fashion jeans under $70.

H&M (hm.com)

Ridiculously inexpensive but trendy, so be picky. Merchandise moves fast so it's hit or miss but go in that spirit. The payoff could be a hot-off-the-runway-looking blazer in a color-of-the-minute. It's a good resource for fast fillers like a **classic faux leather tote, avaiators, belts, scarves, and earrings.** Winter brings out sophisticated parkas that don't look frumpy and slim tunic length sweaters. Check out designer collaborations that pop up and sell out overnight.

J.Crew (jcrew.com)

A candy store of color that suits us. Their neutrals are pitch-perfect and never look dull, dirty, or off. The perfect fit V-neck and ballet-neck tees show exactly the right amount of chest and not cleavage. **The amazing range of cashmere sweaters would be triple the price elsewhere**, and the medium-rise cropped capris and Minnie pants could not make us happier . . . except for the Italian leather ballet flats in every color.

J.Jill (jjill.com)

Everyday basics make this brand age-appropriate in a good way. Everything is scaled to proportions rather than size and available in misses, petites, women's, or tall range. I love the **Wearever line of jersey sheaths, wrap-look skirts, cropped jackets, and wrap dresses with draped and pleated details.** The Pure Jill Kimono sleeve sweaters, work skimmers, loafer flats, stretch cotton slim ankle cropped pants—love all!

Kmart (kmart.com)

Check the Jaclyn Smith line for extremely low-cost basics like knee-length pencils and blazers. **You'll find classic pea coats, hooded toggle coats, and puffers all under $100.**

Kohl's (kohls.com)

Vera Wang's Simply Vera collection is for us. **You want Vera's feminine cardigans and tops with beading and tulle** in her signature soft grey and browns—and her sunglasses and flats.

L.L. Bean (llbean.com)

Certain outdoorsy items here have a sexy Euro-chic look. The **water-resistant quilted vests and riding jackets** are lean and fit to wear with leggings or slim jeans and Bean's Wellies or shearling boots—all great low-priced alternatives to more fashion-y brands.

Lands' End (landsend.com)

Get their **ponte knits, perfect no iron shirts,** white cotton and chambray tunics to pair with slim pants or jeans, metallic parkas in gold and silver, driving mocs, and driving mules.

Levi's (levi.com)

Yes, the **Curve ID jeans system** really works, but I prefer the Heritage Fits collection that includes the 505 straight-leg cut. Levi's rises won't make you squirm and are all in the $50 range. Their boyfriend jeans are a must-get for a relaxed look but these go fast so shop online.

Talbots (talbots.com)

For conservative classics in sizes 12 to 24W and petite 12 to 22 that suit a conservative office or traditional workplace, this is the source. Beautiful dresses and slim cropped pants.

Target (target.com)

You need to cherry-pick but hang in there to find **lightweight jersey knit dresses, decorative flats, water-repellent trenches, and men's pajamas and robes** that look sexy and cool on us.

Liz Lange for Target maternity dresses are contemporary for 40+ moms who are also saving their splurges for a post-baby personal trainer and Botox.

The Outnet (outnet.com)

This discount site by the very luxurious Net-A-Porter retail site offers **wildly reduced designer clothing**, pop up sales, and going going gone sales. Pick up a Helmut Lang satin trench reduced from $650 to $292 or a Sonia Rykiel bag reduced from $765 to $230.

Uniqlo (uniqlo.com)

This low-cost Japanese retailer has modern clean-lined basics with a sleek shape and proportions. Don't miss the **super-light down jackets, tunics, and tees**.

Victoria's Secret (victoriassecret.com)

Never mind bras and panties, the **sweaters and tops** you can order online are a best-kept secret.

Wal-Mart (walmart.com)

Snap up **basic black fillers** like opaque tights, long sleeve tees, camisoles, jersey wrap robes, simple chemise nightgowns, and jersey dresses—all in your fave neutral.

White House Black Market (whitehouseblackmarket.com)

Everything is black and white. The **pencils, ponte pieces, sleeveless tailored dresses, and draped tops** make a stop worth it.

Zara (zara.com)

They have plenty of well-fitting contemporary tailored clothes but watch the skirt/dress length. The **blazers, overcoats, dresses, and blouses are fabulous** but don't skip the men's department. I find scarves, hats, sweaters, and tees here too all the time. Merchandise changes quickly so buy it when you see it.

CHAPTER THREE

I WANNA BE ME…STICK WITH YOUR OWN LOOK!

We're a generation of rule-breakers and original thinkers.

Personal style—in the real, everyday people sense—is a concept that was created and encouraged by fashion magazines. There was genuine reasoning and marketing behind this idea. Editors and advertisers discovered that by using celebs and actresses as fashion "role models" and creating style categories, women more easily identified with trends and shopped with a greater sense of urgency.

"Get the _____ look" is still a potent editorial strategy in print and on-line. But by 40 every woman knows she is the star of her own life. We're not really influenced that much by what celebrities wear—even those who are our peers. Most of us don't look at women in their twenties and thirties either. And although we love historic fashion icons—the Hepburns, Coco Chanel, and Jackie —we don't want to dress like them . . . at least not anymore. We're only interested in "that's me!" or "that's not me!"

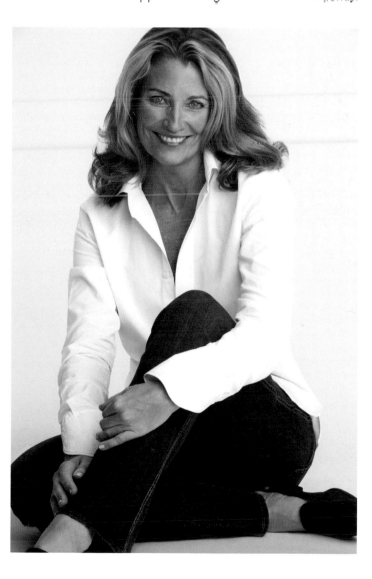

Patricia Neville

Here's the real backstory

There was a time when women got their fashion inspiration looking at high-end fashion magazines that featured a small group of very creative models who actually did inspire trends. There were no stylists and no brands or labels controlling the editorial decisions. Now actresses, rock stars, celeb-models, and C-list reality TV stars all dressed by stylists (who think of themselves as celebrities, too) have bumped everyday models off magazine covers. In the late '60s and early '70s models did their own hair and makeup (or at least played a big part in the creation). They also brought their lives, interests, and style chops straight into the studio, where they participated in creating the photos. These models shaped the way we dress and think about clothes. They include:

Model icon and celebrity/beauty entrepreneur **Lauren Hutton**—the first to combine a jean skirt, a man's white shirt, and Converse sneakers as a uniform.

Super-natural supermodel **Cheryl Tiegs,** who put beachy California style on our radar.

Supermodel **Marisa Berenson,** the first model to do bohemian style.

Jerry Hall and **Janice Dickinson** gave us lessons in glamour.

Patti Hansen and **Paulina Porizkova** made edgy okay and achievable.

'60s icon **Twiggy** made us believe in the power of a simple shift dress, tights, and flats.

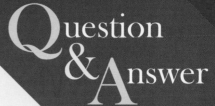

Q: What's YOUR style?

A: Style? I just buy what I like.

Most fashion books and magazines categorize women in weird groupings with names like artsy, rocker, bohemian, bombshell, gamine—whatever, we don't get it. Ask any woman over 40 what her current style is and she'll most likely pause and not have an immediate answer. You can push and say, "Would you call yourself trendy?" She'll think a minute and then say, "No, not really." We don't think of ourselves in terms of what we wear; we think of ourselves according to how we live. Most women I interviewed for this book used words like "simple, classic, comfortable" to describe her style. My fashion categories are a little more reality-based and reflect the way we think and feel about clothes, our bodies, and our multi-level lifestyles now.

What a fashion update can do for you now

I wouldn't dare try to tell you to change your personal taste, so my biggest piece of advice is this: stay fluid. Like us, fashion is always a work in progress—renewing, improving, updating, and refreshing itself. We're an experimental group of women; we're independent thinkers who are comfortable with change.

We update our faces with Botox, fillers, lasers, wrinkle-smoothing creams, facelifts, and lasers to erase age spots and sun damage. We have tooth-whitening visits to the dentist. So we want problem-solving underwear and de-aging clothes solutions, too!

We renew our cars for our new lives with fuel-efficient hybrids, easy-park Mini Coopers, and snappy two-seater convertibles now that the kids are grown. So we want edited wardrobes that are modern and efficient also.

We rethink the concept of home and trade family homes for manageable condos and work-free townhouses. So we want less but better, affordable but stylish fashion, too.

We upgrade our personal electronic gadgets and have the latest cell phones, juicers, sonic face scrubbers, electric toothbrushes, blow-dryers, and flatirons. So we want improved fabrics and multi-purpose, seasonless style.

Knowing when to change and move your shopping habits to the next level is also part of the process. Don't look back.

Me too! Same thing!

I have always been a little rebellious when it comes to style. First day on the job as beauty and fashion director of *Ladies' Home Journal* the entire editorial staff, including myself, was whisked off to a sales meeting in Bermuda. I was expected to speak about my plans for our new and improved fashion coverage. Everyone was dressed in '80s dress-for-success corporate casual—tailored jackets and conservative business attire with sheer hose. What did I wear? A black leather pencil skirt from agnès b. with a crisply ironed white Hanes boy's T-shirt, bare legs, and possibly no bra. Fresh out of the box from the groovier environment of *Mademoiselle* magazine, I simply wore (what was for me anyway) a typical work look. I continued to dress for my career as a fashion editor in my own quirky way, working my way through designer labels and trends but sticking to the things that made me happy. Leather pencil skirts and Hanes boy's tees are still on my list. So are vintage jeans and cowboy boots. I love fashion but I love wearing clothes that suit me even more.

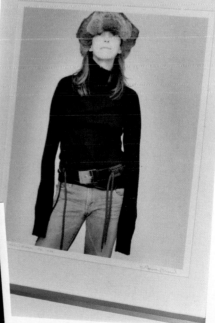

About 2005, wearing my trapper, jeans, and black turtle winter uniform

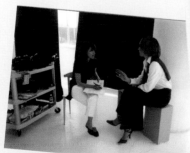

At the studio interviewing a MORE reader

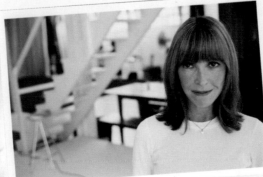

In 2003, photographed by Arthur Elgort for makeup guru Sonia Kashuk's book "Real Beauty"

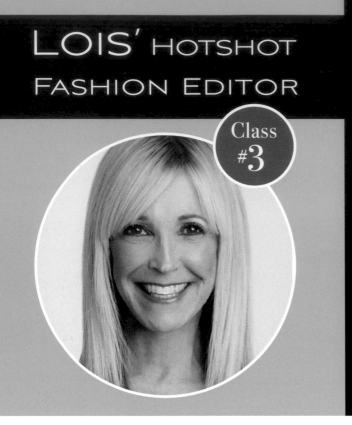

Class
#3

10 No-Fail Booster Tricks, Whatever Your Style

1. Sit like a front-row celeb, stand like a model. Your personal body language helps or hurts the way you look in clothes. This is especially true after 40, when bone mass starts to go, muscles sag, and fat creeps up on us. Working with thousands of real women on photo shoots, my biggest fashion issue was teaching women to move with ease and body awareness. The major difference between models or celebrities and real women

as they age is this: pros compensate for body flaws in front of the camera or a crowd. You don't need to pose; just be more aware of posture and how you move. Ready for a shock? Check out grown-up, sophisticated women as they walk down the street or sit in restaurants. Some of those dressed-to-kill fashionistas slump, slouch, and lumber. You think they'd know money can't buy everything.

> An amazing wardrobe, a healthy body, and astonishing charisma don't do a thing if you can't stand, sit, and walk with grace. It's never too late to learn. Here are the main things to know:

- **Walking:** Walk tall. Step on the ball of the foot and roll to the toes. If you're wearing heels, make sure your shoes have a cushy liner like Foot Petals insoles so you glide, not stomp. Put one foot in front of the other, not side to side. You don't need to mimic the runway strut of a model; just don't lurch.

- **Sitting:** When you're seated and your legs are visible to all (not at the movies, but at a party or in photos, for example) please do cross your legs. Yeah I know it's bad for circulation but it looks sexy, focuses all attention on your face and legs, and makes everything in between (including sag and flab) not count for the moment. Slant both legs after crossing them in the direction of the lower leg (if you cross left over right, slant to your right, and vice versa). Lift the upper leg slightly higher so the calf doesn't bulge out when pressed against the bottom leg.

- **Standing still:** When standing, keep your chin up, neck elongated, shoulders down and back. Lift your rib cage off your hips (imagine a string going all through your body head to toes), keep your stomach tucked in, chest out, and put your weight on one straight leg and bend the other.

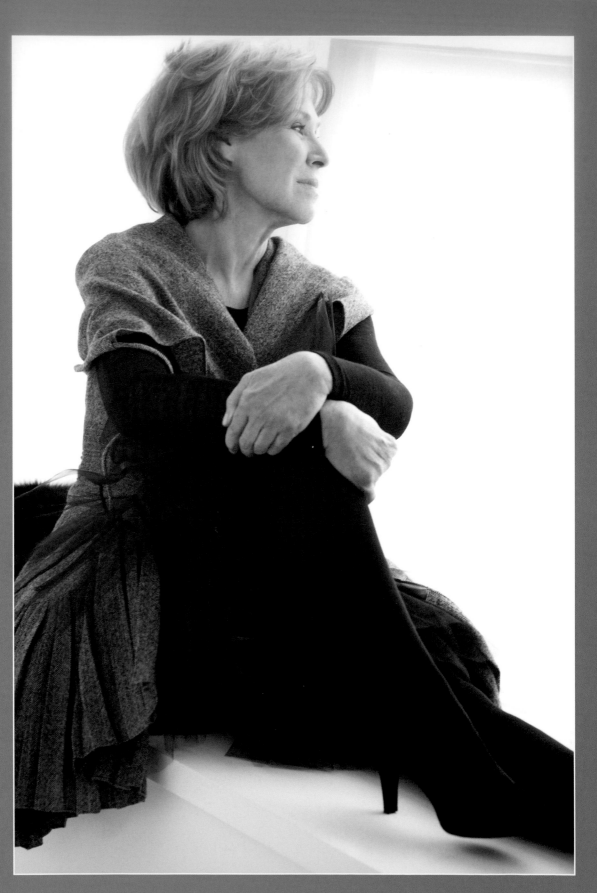

Rule breaker
Jo Gaynor
in Morgane
Le Fay tweed
dress with tulle
crinoline and
peep-toes

2. Consider your shape first, trends second.

Keep that "me first" attitude. How can it possibly work otherwise? Your shape and the shape it's in—your skin tone and personal preferences—influence how clothes perform on your body and in your life.

Not every color, trend, style, or accessory works for every woman. Understand that and you'll never make mistakes.

If you think platform boots or booties look clunky and make your legs look chunky don't wear them. Stay strong and just say no.

3. Keep it seasonless.

Most things we buy from now on should be really versatile, with the exception of cold-weather coats and serious cold-weather boots. The layering concept, improved fabric blends and unpredictable weather (indoors and out) make getting dressed not so different whether we live in Boca Raton or Boston. Modern life itself mixes up the seasons. Offices, planes, and restaurants are alternately freezing, cold, or steamy whether it's June or January. Movie theaters and malls are over air conditioned all summer, spa-like in December. The ultimate solution: blended fabrics that are not too heavy or too light, clothes that work with boots or sandals, pieces that layer on or off easily, and a core wardrobe of neutral colors that look right any place and any time of year.

Ten chic, seasonless essentials are:

1. **Cropped jeans or slim cropped pants:** That work with sweaters or black tees, cropped boots or flip-flops

2. **Classic tan trench coat:** Over skirts or pants, bare legs or tights, a jersey dress or sequins

3. **Long tanks:** To layer and fill gaps

4. **Dark neutral pencil skirt:** In viscose/polyester or ponte for work or evenings twelve months a year

5. **Cotton/cashmere V-necks:** To stretch your neck and pair with matching bottoms

6. **Nude shoes and boots:** To elongate your legs and wear with anything

7. **Fresh white cotton shirt:** To brighten any look in rain, snow, after dark, or when you feel drab

8. **Tailored, body-skimming dress:** For any serious/work/dress-up situation

9. **Three-quarter sleeve cardigans:** The ultimate climate control item to throw on or throw off as needed

10. **Dressy, opaque top with sleeves:** Draped or sequined to glam up pencils, jeans, and pants without the need for layers

4. Break the rules.

Wear leather leggings with a tunic sweater or a zebra print dress to work if that's who you are. It takes fashion guts and a dash of creativity at 40+ to: cinch a vintage army jacket over a businesslike tweed tailored dress, wear orange silk crepe pants with a fuchsia V-neck, or show up in a body-con Hervé Léger dress at your college reunion. If that's you, congratulations because you're a world-class rule breaker. You have a stand-up comic's knack for taking the ordinary and making it extraordinary. All you really need is one amazing visual punch line. It can be something truly simple, like adding a bright yellow bag to a black outfit or wearing a shocking pink coat in winter. If you have the confidence, why not?

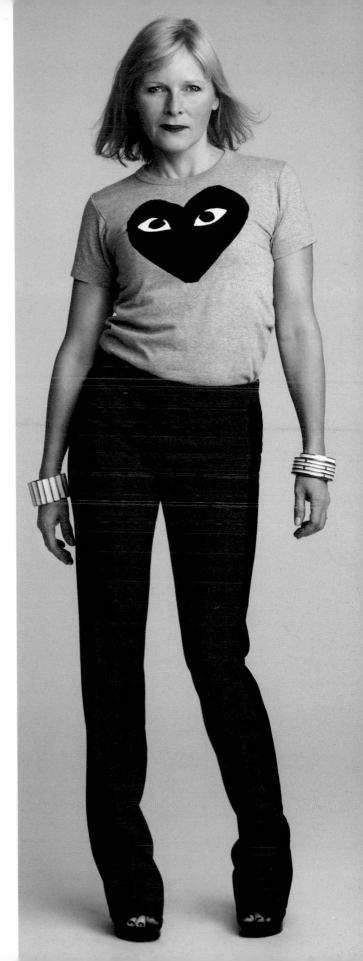

Annemarie Iverson in rule breaker Derek Lam red pants and heart tee from J.Crew

5. Get in shape any way you can.

Get your body into a comfort zone that makes you clothes-happy. You don't have to be thin at all; but let's face it, a firm body does increase your clothes options. If you wear leggings or tight jeans without a second thought or stroll down the beach in a swimsuit and no pareo, you're probably feeling fit and fearless. Otherwise, evaluate your nutrition and step up the exercise just to keep things solid. Self-conscious about your legs? Run on the treadmill, get them waxed, do self-tanner, and buy great nude shoes. Inhibited by your torso? Suck it all in with shapewear, increase your crunches, and wear one-piece dresses.

6. Last-minute fashion fixes work for everyone.

We live and dress at high speed. Everything is so last minute that most women spend five minutes max deciding what to wear. Once we're dressed, who wants to start over or even has the time? E-mail invites and spur-of-the-moment schedule changes don't take no for an answer. We end up running out the door and worrying we look boring, basic, or blah. Add at least one item from list A, one from list B, and you can't miss:

A: Serious heels, a skinny belt, chic eyeglasses

B: A shirt or blouse in an unexpected color or print, a bag in a contrast color, a wow necklace

7. Do the new sexy. It's not about cleavage, minis, or stilettos anymore.

One of the advantages of age is knowing how to be subtle but effective. Here's what's really sexy after 40 now:

Showing bare shoulders or arms: Instead of boobs and thighs

Playing up curves with belts and knits: Instead of tight clingy clothes

Wearing peep-toes or sandals with a trendy pedicure color: Instead of balancing on stilettos

Looking casually cool in our jeans: Instead of minis

Wearing boots and sunglasses for attitude: Instead of designer logos

And don't forget to flash a warm white-toothed smile often, and balance fashion fanaticism with volunteer work and mentoring. That's sexy, too.

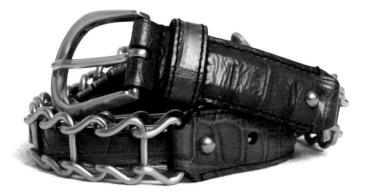

8. Acknowledge your inner superstar/diva/rock star.

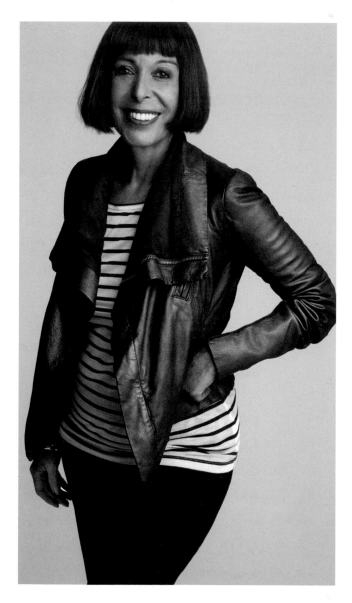

We all have a little Madonna, Halle Berry, or Sharon Stone in us. We can channel our inner diva with dark neutral clothes and one or two superstar elements. Start with a dark body-skimming base. Then add one or two (not more!) of these:

- **Edgy boots:** Over-the-knee, motorcycle, or to-the-knee-high-heel boots

- **Something leather, python, fur, or metallic:** Like a cropped leather jacket or python ankle boots

- **Dramatic inky colors:** Like charcoal, indigo, forest green, and black violet in a scarf, fitted sweater, or nail polish

- **Bold jewels:** Like an oversized ring, statement cuffs, or a chunky multi-chain necklace

Gloria Appel in Rick Owen leather jacket, jeans, and boatneck

9. Vary the fit and mix proportions.

When designers, editors, and stylists are putting together looks, they usually combine fits to vary the proportions. This contrast creates a more interesting dynamic. It's why wearing slouchy boyfriend jeans with a fitted top, a sheath dress under a swingy cropped jacket, or an A-shape tunic over leggings works so well. All clothes fall into one of three fit categories. They're either:

- **Snug and body hugging:** Like leggings, skinny jeans, bodysuits, and stretch turtlenecks

- **Skimming your body but not tight:** Like tailored shirts, slim sweaters and tees, pencil skirts, and sheaths

- **Loose and generously cut:** Like tunics, relaxed jeans and sweaters, silk blouses, and trapeze jackets

10. Go for feel-good fabrics.

We've learned to live in a tech-centric world connected by computer screens, iPhones, and iPads. But our generation is really hardwired for a physical world that's a lot more touchy-feely. We still like in-person face time, eye-to-eye communication, and the pleasurable feeling of fabrics against skin. If we can't have the first two, the third is certainly attainable. Make fashion a totally sensual experience by purposely choosing fabrics that feel good. You can't ignore the softness of vintage jeans, broken in cords, and freshly washed cotton T-shirts.

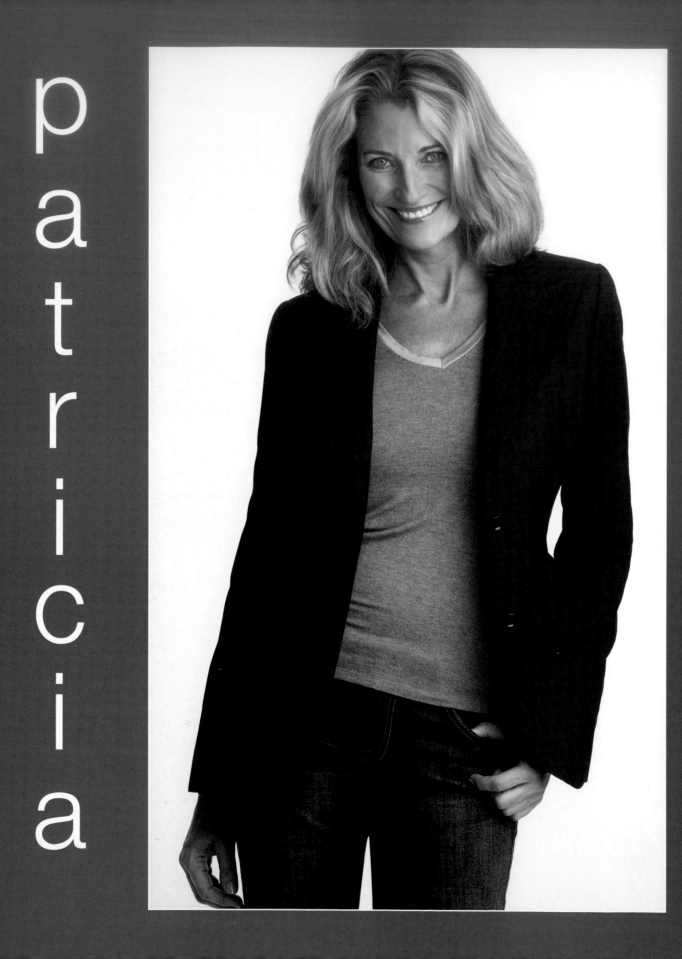

p
a
t
r
i
c
i
a

patricia on:

inspiration: "I'm not willing to be uncomfortable for the sake of fashion. Although I get the opportunity to wear new trends in my work as a model, it doesn't necessarily carry over into my personal wardrobe choices. Comfort is now a necessity, not a perk."

wardrobe: "A white Charvet shirt tailored for me in Paris is by far the most useful, versatile item in my closet. I wear it with everything from jeans to a classic A-line skirt. I edit my clothes down every year and donate whatever doesn't fit my lifestyle any longer. It's quite freeing to have fewer options but quality choices. My diamond studs and Baume & Mercier watch are consistent pieces in my daily wardrobe."

patricia neville

Model, Wilhelmina Agency

TRADE SECRETS

If you live in jeans, are always on a diet, like a little sex appeal with your style, insist on comfort, love looking at trends, or still have a label fetish, you're in good company. Here are ways to update your look and still be you.

THE JEANS FAN

VINTAGE WASHES AND BOYFRIEND STYLES OR TIGHT FASHION JEANS TOP YOUR DAILY "DO" LIST.

Okay! You have a casual, dress-down life and love never having to wear a skirt or dress—even for work. Knowing which jeans to choose is key. Despite all the hype of the jeans industry there are only two jeans: relaxed or tight. Some women like tight stretch "fashion" jeans for the feeling of compression and say it makes them feel slimmer. If this is you, what I call "show-off" jeans that accent your body from the waist down are probably your favorites. These are tight or at least curve hugging and may be bootcut, skinny, or cropped. The rise should be at least a medium style for no belly ledge or bulges at the sides.

Other women love the look and feel of relaxed jeans or prefer to not focus attention on below the waist body issues. A looser, slouchier fit, like a boyfriend or straight leg classic jean, works for them every time. Looser jeans should sit slightly lower than the waist or at the top of the hip (not around your bikini line, so avoid low rises!) and be worn with a belt to define the body. A jeans-only lifestyle still provides an ideal base for infinite fashion possibilities. You can start with a tank or bodysuit. Add a blazer or cropped jacket, a silk blouse, a fitted sweater, and shoes with a heel for elegance. Add a tunic or slouchy layers and flats for ease.

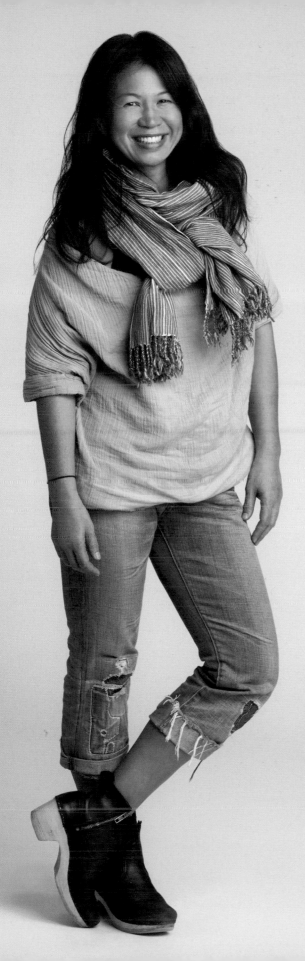

Nikki Wang in boyfriend jeans, casual layers, and clog boots

THE BABE
(BUT I'M NOT A COUGAR!)

So you like looking a little sexy? Whether dating, happily married, or reveling in their single-hood, some women like to be foxy. If you've already ditched flesh-revealing clothes for shape-accenting ones you're on the right track. Keep your allure going in body-skimming sheaths, pencil skirts, slim pants, and fitted tops but refine your use of color and accessories.

MAKE THREE CHANGES:

• **Wear feminine colors in skin-enhancing shades.** Soft coral, apricot, rose pink, and nudes look provocative without being pushy.

• **Make belts your #1 go-to accessory.** They play up your shape and strengthen the hourglass effect in one simple move.

• **Wear nude slingbacks with a tapered toe to stretch your legs.** Heels show off legs but they don't have to be super-high to be effective.

THE CLASSIC
(BUT I'M NOT STUFFY!)

Slip in preppy hipster items like bold framed "nerd" glasses, vintage prints and plaids, and a slightly imperfect attitude. You probably started out preppy with an Ivy League inspiration and then grew into Ralph Lauren land. Now your biggest fear is turning into your mother. Some women still love nothing better than a good pantsuit, crisp button-down shirts, cabled sweaters, and khakis. No problem. Classic always looks cool if you tweak the proportions, combine more relaxed pieces with "starchy" ones, and wear your clothes a little more irreverently.

HERE'S HOW TO TAKE THE STUFFINESS OUT OF TWO CLASSIC LOOKS:

• **To loosen up a classic urban look:** Layer a tank under your shirt, then casually half-tuck the shirt, add a light V-neck sweater or cardigan, and finally the blazer. Pull out the shirt cuffs and roll or flip them up over the jacket sleeves, which should be pushed back. Add slim dark jeans or khakis and your choice of driving shoes or ballet flats, plus big black or tortoise shell sunglasses (the so-called nerd glasses), your favorite hoops and bangles, and structured bag.

• **To update a classic suburban/country/weekend look:** Layer a tank, shirt, or V-neck; add slim broken-in khakis or vintage wash jeans. Add a waxed jacket or quilted vest, driving shoes or Converse sneakers, and a hobo or messenger bag. You get my drift? The idea is not to change your style but to refresh it. Do a hoodie instead of a V-neck for example, but the overall strategy is the same. Keep your classic raincoats, polos, pleated skirts, and your monogrammed L.L. Bean canvas tote—can't mess with perfection.

THE YO-YO DRESSER

No one suits one-color dressing more than you. Make it your mantra. You have rarely stayed the same weight for an entire year and your closet tells your story. Size 6, 8, 10, and 14? You are probably a lifelong dieter who has "skinny clothes" and more forgiving ones. The key to staying fashionable now is to not concentrate on a size or have a "When I lose the weight philosophy . . ." Now you need to be sure the pieces you wear the most have built-in flexibility to compensate for weight fluctuations.

THESE ARE THREE THINGS YOU CAN DO NOW TO MAKE FASHION FUN AND FLATTERING:

• **Make ponte knits a priority:** Ponte is a thick, double knit that's stretchy enough to accommodate extra curves yet has enough structure to whittle a clean sharp silhouette. Choose slim, body-skimming styles rather than those that are oversized or too roomy. Try ponte in pants, pencils, dresses, skirts, tunics, and jackets.

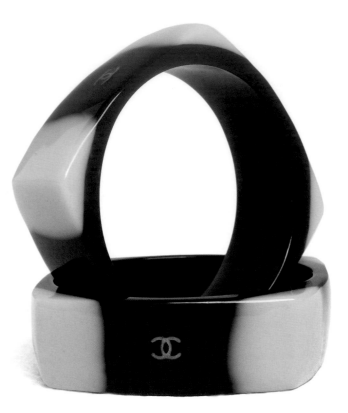

- Continue to work the one-color matching and toning strategy (per Chapter 1): And focus attention on elongating and lengthening your body with open necklines and shoes that help create the illusion of longer legs. Where does the fun come in? Have you ever been to the Uffizi Gallery in Florence or the Louvre in Paris? Those sixteenth- and seventeenth-century babes were not a size 2 and knew how to work a one-color look with jewels better than anyone.

- Make jewelry your big splurge item. Collect statement necklaces and bracelets. They don't have to be real or even costly costume. Finding great junk jewelry at flea markets, online sites, and consignment shops is a sport all by itself—and a great distraction from Ben & Jerry's Schweddy Balls.

THE LABEL LOVER

GET STREET-Y AND MIX MALL HAULS WITH MAJOR DESIGNER PIECES. Confess. You're the type who may not say, "Whose is it?" out loud anymore but it's still the first thing you think. Your closet is probably a museum of designer clothes and accessories, including those from the '80s and '90s still in their original garment bags and boxes. Don't be show-y now but don't be shy either. Just mix it up more. Wear luxurious items you love (even those that scream designer with logos and recognizable features that pinpoint the era) with low-key casual ones and new pieces picked up at the mall. Letting go of status gives you more space to play with clothes in a modern, contemporary way and re-energize the items you have.

THE COMFORT QUEEN

I hear you. You're always too hot or too cold and menopause makes you feel like aliens from the planet Bloat have taken over your body. At some point for many women, comfort is no longer negotiable; in fact it comes before any other style criteria. My advice is to add soothers—those pieces that make fashion enjoyable again and delete the irritants you can't ignore. Editing your closet is first on the agenda. Soft dressing—knits and sweaters rather than structured clothes—will probably be the basis of your entire wardrobe. Look for stretch in everything from microfiber pull-on boots to your weekend tees.

HERE ARE THE TEN MOST COMFORTABLE ITEMS TO WEAR:

1. Relaxed or boyfriend-style jeans

2. Seamless T-back bras

3. Seamless girl-short panties

4. Camisoles with built-in bras

5. Lightweight nylon bags

6. Relaxed tanks and tees

7. Soft cowl, V, and ballet necklines

8. Raglan sleeve sweaters and coats

9. Driving shoes

10. Shearling lined boots—yes, like UGG boots, which I happen to think are great!

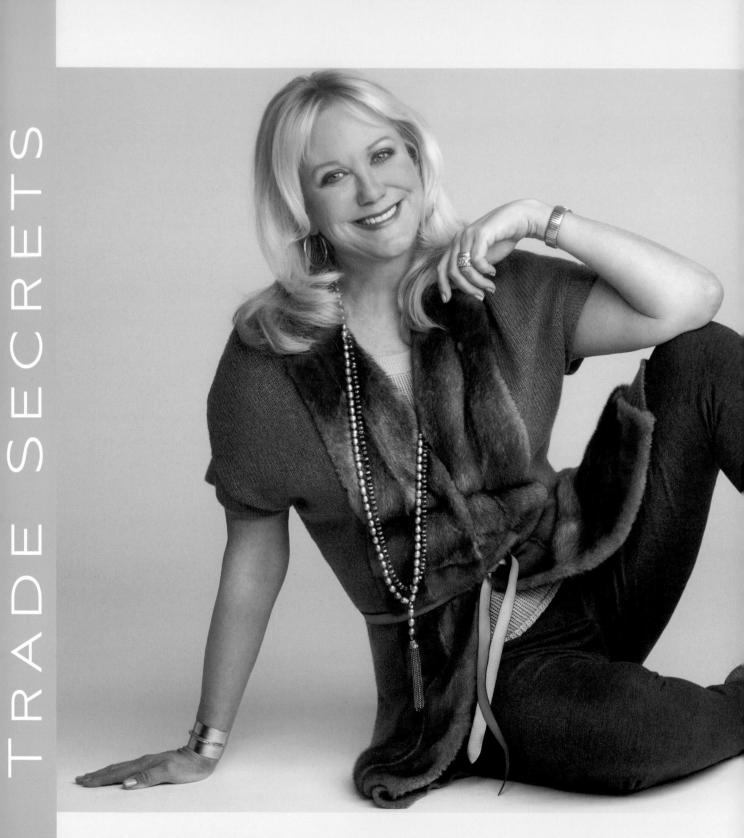

THE TREND-ISTA

New fashion trends recharge your style battery. Who says you can't wear them all? You can still be trendy after 40, but be selective so the clothes don't appear to be wearing you.

YOU HAVE THREE CHOICES WHEN IT COMES TO TRENDS:

- **If you like the look or thrill of trends head-to-toe:** Select the tamest version instead of the most extreme. These items just may have an afterlife in your wardrobe when they die out on the runway and in the fashion pages.

- **If you are craving a specific trendy color, fabric, or detail:** Get one item that will work with all your neutrals as an accent and update. This way you don't look like a fashion victim.

- **If you want a super-trendy, very youthful item:** Buy it low-cost so you won't kick yourself a month later when you wish you hadn't.

Trend-ista Nina Griscom
in fur booties and vest

TRADE SECRETS

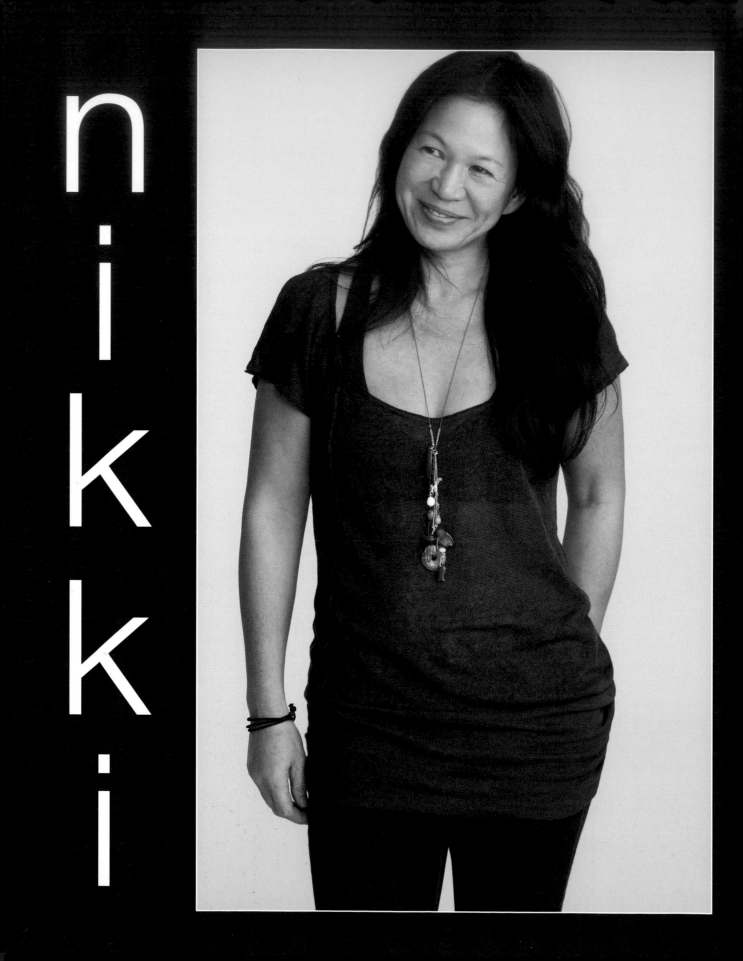

n
i
k
k
i

nikki on:

style: "My style is basically relaxed but has changed to a more athletic and ethnic-inspired one. Since I've started Thai boxing and Brazilian Jiu-Jitsu my feet are wider and don't fit into fancy shoes. I prefer bold colors and lots of texture and use scarves to accent everything from jeans to dresses and adjust my clothes to temperature changes."

age and fashion: "I still wear shorts but maybe I should stop soon since I'm 46! But I love my strong legs and at 5'2" I can get away with shorter lengths. My big tricks are to wear more open necklines, and a tighter fit around the torso (it makes everyone look taller and slimmer). I see trying to cover any un-flattering parts of my body as a kindness to the public! But at the same time my attitude is, wear whatever makes you feel good. When I dress I'm not really conscious of what other people will think, to be honest."

nikki wang

Sculptor, freelance makeup artist

I'm Obsessed with . . .

Let's admit it. Sure we're interested and involved in the bigger issues like politics, world stability, finance, environmental changes, health care, and unemployment, but we still love to check out how other women put themselves together. This doesn't make us superficial; it makes us consistent. We can't help admiring our sisters in style.

If you think about:

How other women my age dress: Go on and be a voyeur. Take a look at what they do and figure out what attracts or intrigues you most about their clothes. Is it the technique of dressing: the way they accessorize, tie a scarf, layer, combine unexpected pieces or use color? Is the attraction due to the pieces themselves? A certain neckline or the fit of a jacket? Think about what these women do to give ordinary clothes a stylish twist. Then adapt their look into your own way of putting clothes together.

Keeping my look consistent: Women with a distinctive personal style make choices. They don't try to wear everything on the fashion menu. You really can't be all over the place after 40. Stick to what works for you and own it. Then play with color, shape, layers and subtle updates. Each of us has a favorite basic look at this point. For me it's skinny jeans, boots, and a black cashmere sweater.

looking at My Peers.

Buying fakes: Sorry but one sad fact of fashion is seen on the streets of big cities and in small boutiques and salons that sell accessories on the side: phony designer bags complete with knock-off logos, shapes, and prints. Aside from the illegality of selling fakes I have an issue with women buying wannabes. Buy the best bag you can afford and don't try to look richer, cooler, more successful, or fashionable with a faux, because you won't.

Wearing the same pieces over and over: Having the fashion smarts to buy versatile pieces you can wear a hundred different ways is the sign of style wisdom. In fact, lots of fashion pros repeat the same pieces two or three times a week and never wear them the same way twice. This is how investment items of great quality pay for themselves. It's also why buying multiples of perfect low-cost basics when you find them is the right thing to do.

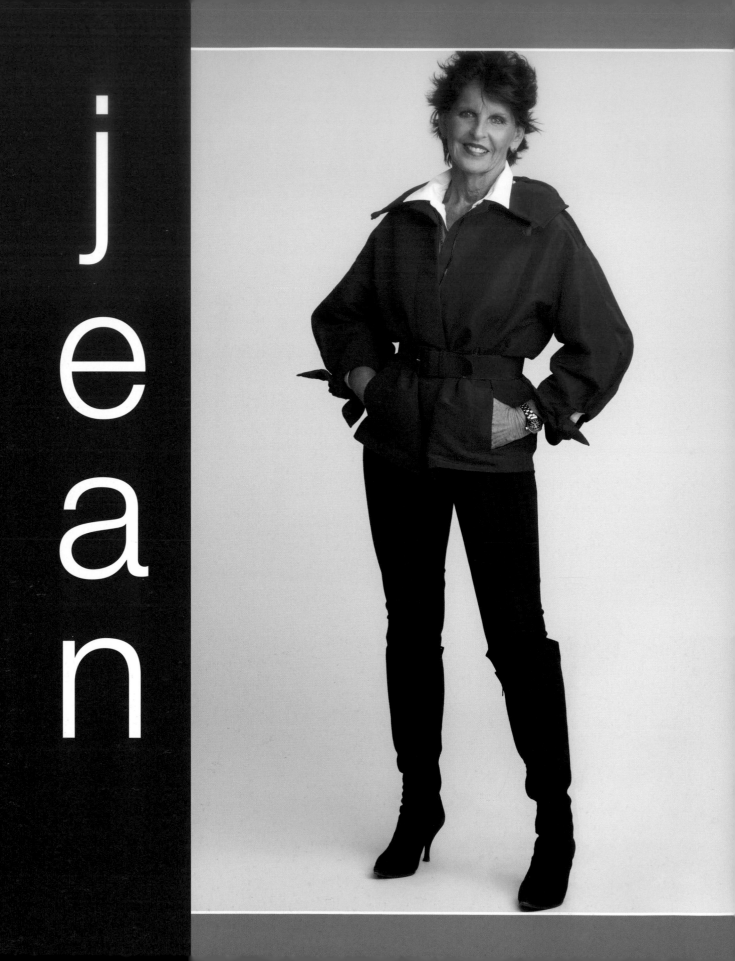

jean

jean on:

style: "Photos of me from every decade reveal the same fashion loves—white shirts, jeans, classic jackets, and boots. I've always liked specific colors, especially black, strong blues and reds, beige, and white. However, over the last five years two things have influenced the way I dress and my fashion needs: a switch from a full-time, six days a week career to my own part-time consulting business and a bout with breast cancer. The latter left me cancer-free today but with one arm about three inches larger than the other due to post-surgery lymphodema. I like to be more covered up so it's not as noticeable (so sad to shelve those sleeveless shirts). I do consulting for Oscar de la Renta and the office is full of smart young women with a style that's inspiring. I pay more attention to accessories, especially scarves. And I'm definitely influenced by Oscar's wonderful sense of color and use of elaborate fabrics and prints. As I went through chemo I learned to dress in layers for comfort and to use scarves creatively. Those styling tricks have stayed with me."

jean hoehn zimmerman

The Top Style Mistakes Women Make

Wearing what you like best is not the end of the story. Personal style still benefits from a few straightforward guidelines.

LET'S AGREE NOT TO DO THIS ANYMORE:

1. **Wear leather too aggressively.** Combine leather with soft or feminine pieces. There's a good reason editors and stylists usually pair more refined pieces with leather: because otherwise the look is just too tough. I love my black leather Belstaff motorcycle jacket and wear it with leggings and boots, but it looks drop-dead chic with a slim black pencil skirt.

2. **Buy one-note clothes.** Go for maximum versatility. Convertible fashion offers quick change, functional solutions.

HERE ARE SOME OF MY FAVORITE TIME-SAVERS:

- **Dual color tights:** Like the SPANX Tight-End Tights Reversible (SPANX.com) that reverse from black to charcoal

- **Super-light down jackets:** Like those by the Japanese brand Uniqlo (uniqlo.com) work as liners for any coat or jacket or on their own

- **Multi-way dresses:** That transform ten ways, like those by Victoria's Secret for the beach and resort vacations (victoriassecret.com)

- **Long drape-front cardigans that wrap many ways:** Like the DKNY long sleeve cozy (dkny.com)

- **Bags that convert from shoulder bag to tote:** Like the Michael Kors Hamilton (michaelkors.com) to free up your hands or make adding heavier items throughout the day easy

- **Rubber Wellies with cozy washable liners:** Like those by Hunter (hunter.com) for hygiene and comfort

3. **Wear clothes that are too darn tight.** A second-skin fit is great for layering pieces, tights, shapewear, undies, swimsuits, and leggings. But when jeans and knits, jackets, and skirts reveal bulges, flab, or rolls it's time for a do-over. Either bite the bullet and get into shapewear so the compression tightens and smoothes the way for your existing wardrobe or loosen up and go for a more relaxed fit and layering technique in the way you dress.

4. **Layer when you'd rather not.** Some women are ardent minimalists and believe a top and bottom is about as complicated as clothes should get. For some, partnering a long top with narrow pants is the uniform du jour. The top can be a long body-skimming sweater or an embellished tunic, and the pant might be a white ankle cropped jean but the long-over-narrow proportion makes it tick.

5. **Buy vintage just because it's designer.** Sometimes vintage is frumpy and sometimes its fab. Even famous designers get caught up in the moment and make mistakes, and sometimes certain items would have worked better about a decade ago. Look for pieces that fill gaps in your closet or upgrade basic items you own in fit and fabric.

6. **Overdo the hippie look after 40.** Bohemian style is forever but if your daily look is a long handkerchief hem maxi skirt, tie-dyed tee, fringed bag, masses of beads, and dangly earrings you need to edit. I'd keep the hippie thing going on top and trim down the bottom. Accessories like slouchy boots, hip-grazing belts, a floppy brim hat, and a fringed or embroidered bag are all ideal extras for jeans—just not all at once.

CHAPTER FOUR

AGELESS vs. AGE-APPROPRIATE

Some women like to blur the boundaries of age, others have a clear opinion how grown-ups should look.

Age distortion is the fashionable disease of the decade. Who looks their real age anymore? We're in a tricky sociological moment since dermatological

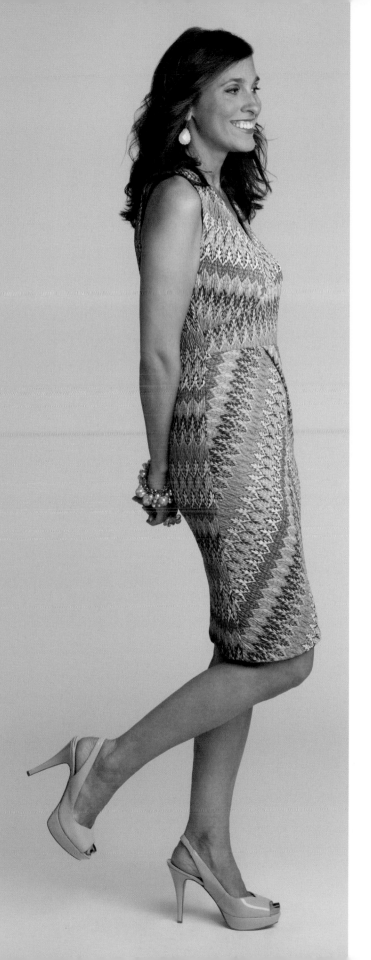

procedures, cosmetic surgery, diets, fitness regimens, hair color, cosmetics, and clothes make it hard to tell if a woman is 45 or 62. Some women boast about their age and are proud of their accomplishments and looks. Others flat-out lie about it (or forget to mention grown children and grandchildren!). Some just refuse to divulge any number at all.

Now that even women in their sixties and seventies are wearing skinny jeans and inky dark nail polish, an ageless, irreverent attitude towards fashion seems to be taking over. Or is it? It seems to me that every woman has her own fashion idea of what's acceptable. So age is not truly as irrelevant as it seems. The age-appropriate topic became fuzzy around the time *Sex and the City* debuted on HBO in 1998. The idea that we could fuse life, work, sex, love, and fashion into one glamorous montage began to seriously seep into our consciousness. Then as Carrie, Charlotte, Samantha, and Miranda aged, so did we.

Hilary Black

Here's the
real backstory

- **The concept of age-appropriate is not really dead.** We realize what we wear has nothing to do with the number of candles on the cake, yet it has everything to do with personal style and the reality of the mirror.

- **There are more similarities between us and younger women than differences these days.** We shop in the same stores, wear a lot of the same brands, have matching hairstyles and buy identical bags and shoes. Our daughters borrow our clothes and vice versa.

- **We're a more diverse group than ever and not that easy to define.** Labeling us based on outdated data is not acceptable. We can be 63 and in incredible shape, 59 and wearing five-inch heels every day, 62 and dating, or 42 and marrying for the first time.

- **If we can't talk, think, walk, sit, and relax in it we'll pass.** Most of us now reject any item of clothing that feels physically or psychologically uncomfortable whether we love the look or not. Our tolerance for discomfort and exposure differs though. Some women think five-inch heels are "normal" everyday shoes and can speed walk through a full workday without a whimper or a blister. Others have fallen for flats and promised unconditional loyalty—no more heels forever.

Q: How do you stay contemporary without looking too young? How do you stay sophisticated without looking stuffy?

A: You need a balance—hot enough to look youthful (but not silly) and fashionable enough to look new (but not desperate). We all have an ageless side that's experimental even if we confine it to food, travel, online dating, or films. Our responsible grown-up side comes in handy in relationships, work, and dealing with all the lemons life throws us. Use that responsible side to evaluate splurges, reason away impulse buys, edit out what's not working anymore, and make new choices based on your life, body, and finances. Use the daring side to try new colors, prints, styles, accessories, brands, and ways to shop. A combo of ageless and age-appropriate is the best possible mix, and we all have varying percentages.

What facing the age issue can do for your clothes now

No matter what our style we all get stuck in fashion ruts. Certain women find safety in serial shopping. They buy and wear the same clothes over and over. This strategy suits some but traps others. They'd benefit from taking a few risks. Other women buy whatever's new and trendy and rarely repeat the same purchases twice. They'd benefit from a base of updated basics and classics to balance their trendier purchases.

Trying on a new-for-you look each season does do one important thing for everyone: It opens your eyes to possibilities. Take a chance either way.

Me too! Same thing! I'm really on the fence here. I'm a grown-up fashion editor who makes practical smart clothing choices but I have an ageless, irreverent attitude about style. As a result my wardrobe has a dual personality. I want the "smart choice" nude sling-backs but I crave the glitter-covered Miu Miu pumps. I need the classic black pencil skirt but I really want the one covered in tiers of tulle. My fashion pro self knows what I should buy and wear but my stylish alter ego can't resist anything that looks like fun.

**Lois in Belstaff biker jacket
and tailored YSL pencil skirt**

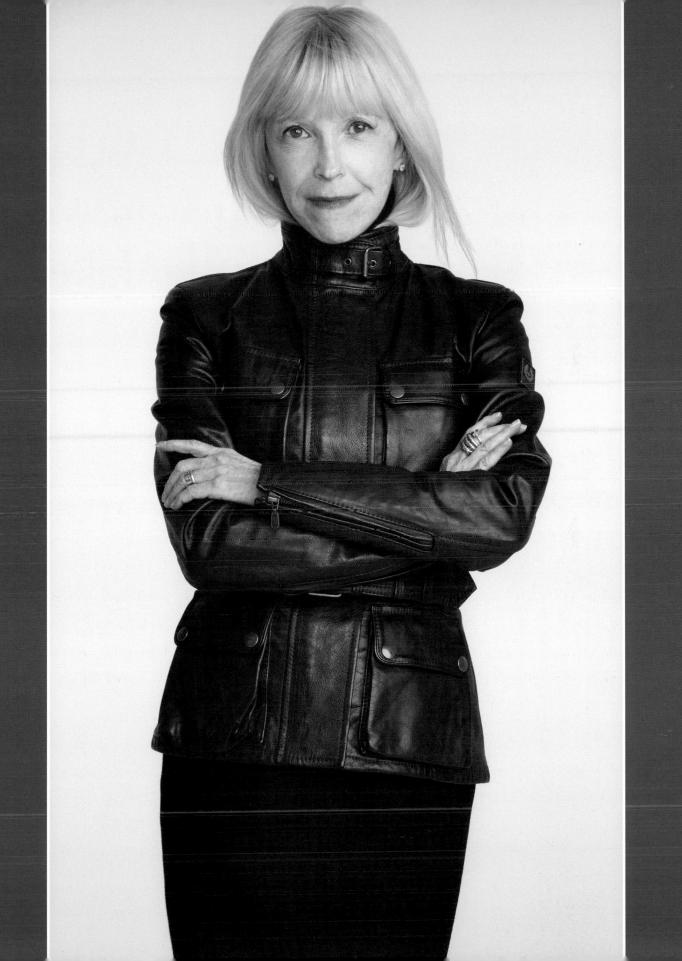

LOIS' HOTSHOT FASHION EDITOR

Class #4

10 Tips
for Looking
Agelessly
Age-Appropriate

1. You can't have it all. Make decisions.

The famous quote "elegance is refusal" belongs to legendary *Vogue* editor Diana Vreeland and Coco Chanel. I agree. Very few women over 40 can pull off extreme fashion. They are nearly always women who work in and around the fashion business and benefit from the attention and paparazzi photos. Real women have to make choices.

How far into fashion your clothes go depends on your body, lifestyle, and your ability to know when enough is enough.

Anyone can wear a chartreuse pencil skirt or a bright green cardigan with beading at the neck or an armful of colorful bangles—but few of us can pull it off all at once.

If you have enough clothes charisma and personal style you probably can—especially if you live in a big city and are in the art, entertainment, music, media, fashion, or public relations world. The rest of us mortals over 40 have to choose. Maybe you'd add the bag and bangles to a neutral dress, or team the skirt with a darker green top or belt the cardigan over a floral print dress.

2. Leopard is our neutral. Wear it naturally.

Back in the '60s, Bond girl Ursula Andress dressed in a leopard coat and boots, and Bob Dylan sang about a leopard hat on his *Blonde on Blonde* album. We never got over it. In fact, we adopted leopard as our "plaid." Animal prints gave us a sexy aura without having to bare a thing and still do. The smallest, spottiest prints—cheetah, leopard, ocelot (and don't attempt to identify which is which)—are feminine and easiest to wear. Larger stripes or boxy patterns like zebra, tiger, and giraffe need a wide flat surface for impact—especially great on bags.

Neutral toned animal prints work with solid black, brown, or tan but mix well with red or orange too. The best animal prints for us are flat matte fabrics in body-skimming sweaters, tailored skirts, blouses, bags, scarves, shoes, coats, belts, and swimsuits. Don't worry about overloading your wardrobe with too many; just wear one major piece or accessory at a time. Here's what not to get: leopard leggings, leopard pantyhose, or leopard jeans. Ever.

> Keep the colors true to those found in nature. After 40, metallic tiger stripes or red and black leopard looks cheesy, even on a swimsuit.

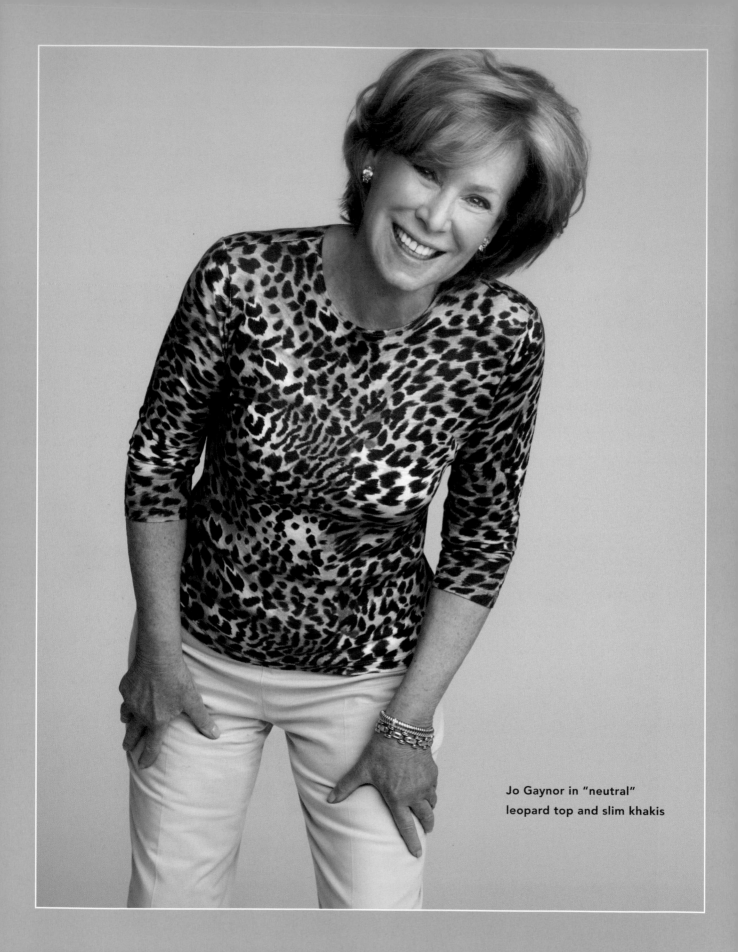

Jo Gaynor in "neutral"
leopard top and slim khakis

3. You can wear anything

with the right underwear.

Who says you can't wear knit skirts or white jeans after 40? It's the underwear, not the clothes that hold you back. I understand the eye appeal of crystal studded or red lace "date" thongs but know this: they are useless. Smooth, seamless microfiber panties may not be showstoppers but they're the next best thing to having a perfect body. For years we've been conditioned to think G-strings and thongs are the ultimate no-bulge, no-bump solution. Well they're not, so let's all come out and say how relieved we are. I've always been super skeptical about the sanitary issue of thongs anyway. Don't tell me this hasn't crossed your mind!

Seamless microfiber briefs don't bind or grab onto fleshier bits at the hip or leg and there is no ick factor.

Choose either a hipster girl-short or a higher, hip-covering boy-short style. The Commando low-rise girl shorts ($26, saksfifthavenue.com, barenecessities.com) in black and nude are the ultimate as far as I'm concerned and are always in my styling kit. Other options by Hanro, Yummie Tummie, and Maidenform may work for you. These or a pair of SPANX shapewear should be enough to get you into anything you want to wear.

4. Dresses are usually better buys than skirts.

Dresses will always be the easier, faster solution anyway. There's no matching or putting together tops and bottoms and no decisions about layers. No matter what style dress you choose—a ladylike sheath, a sporty shift, or shapely knit—the advantages of a one-piece look will always outweigh separates if you have a busy, tightly scheduled lifestyle. Just by adding from a selection of belts, cardigans, jackets, shoes, and bags you push the look from day to night, colorful to neutral, business-like to social, relaxed to serious.

5. Wear knits to solve body problems now.

Classy knits have always been a magnet for grown-up working women. We suspected the blend of style and comfort would get us through long days, meetings, business trips, and commuting crease-free and they did. But despite the love, we knew knits were ultimately going to be trouble. Knit pants sagged at the knees, knit skirts and dresses highlighted tummy, hip, and thigh bulges. Waistbands stretched out and everything bagged around our derriere like a diaper. They made us self-conscious about every jiggle and wiggle. That's all over now.

New firmer knit blends combine stretch and structure, so skirts, pants, and dresses stay in shape.

We've learned a lot from sports performance fabrics. Higher Lycra/spandex content, improved blends, and thicker fabrics with hold make modern knits more durable and comfortable than ever. We can sit, squat, crouch, cross our legs, run up stairs, or dash for a train with total ease and no concerns about looking droopy or lumpy. My own navy and black ponte knit pencils are the most useful versatile skirts I own. Make a ponte pencil your new starter knit piece. Get detail-free clean lines (no pockets, zips, buttons) from brands like J.Jill and Ann Taylor.

6. Really crave color? Buy it in a dress or coat.

Fashion magazines always suggest buying color in an accessory but I think that's a tease. After 40 the flattery of color is sometimes best right next to your skin, where it does the most good. Strategic use of color in your clothes can also help freshen your décolletage, arms, and legs while providing a flattering frame for your face.

> Adding more color to our clothes gives our complexion a real power surge when our skin tone changes due to age, sun damage, or a decision to finally stop tanning.

- **If your skin has gone pale or ashy with age,** energize it with dresses or a coat in vibrant nail polish colors like warm reds, roses, and corals that give it a juicy, youthful look.

- **If your skin is showing its age and sun damage with pigmentation issues** like brown spots, blotchiness, and dark under-eye circles, wearing white, cream, warm nudes, soft pinks, and fruity shades will provide a fresh head-to-toe glow.

- **If your skin has gotten more sallow or ruddy with age,** cool color-saturated blues and purples like plum, midnight blue, cobalt, and fuchsia will counteract any yellow or pink undertones.

- **Don't be afraid to wear strong color head-to-toe** in a monochromatic dress and coat duo, for example. The effect can be shocking—like finally hitting on the right hair color.

7. Decide how much skin to bare or clean it up!

Somewhere along the way we sign a mental nondisclosure agreement with our body. Some women won't show their chest or legs due to brown spots, others won't go sleeveless. It's time to make some definite decisions about how much leg, arm, and cleavage you're willing to display from now on. It will speed up shopping and dressing. Kill an hour waiting for your Boniva to digest by making a list of all the clothes you own that reveal (what you now consider) too much skin. Find solutions for every piece you still want to wear. You may need to rethink your layering, coverage and basics.

Clean up your visible skin (neck, chest, arms, hands, and legs) to free up your clothing choices or make some tough calls about clothes.

You can also see a dermatologist about your options. They may include topical prescription skin care, freezing with cryotherapy, a series of mild chemical peels, or laser. Think about if it's worth it to you in the long run. It may just be.

8. Keep your edge.

Designer Norma Kamali once told me the secret of staying youthful is to stay in touch with your inner girl. Norma (the mother of modern, youthful clothes) meant keep the attitude and energy going and stay curious, open to new things. Fashion is one way to do exactly that. One little shot of daring does it. Edge can be simple as wearing gladiator sandals with a tailored dress, a green leather biker jacket with jeans, and a brilliant purple scarf with everything (all examples straight from the women featured in this book). For me it's bold black glasses, yellow-blonde statement hair that's frankly fake, and my Hermès black leather bracelets and biker jacket.

9. Dress-up and dress-down for the unexpected.

We're the generation that wanted it all and we still do. We want to look contemporary but appropriate, relaxed but authoritative, sophisticated but youthful. Life and personal style don't always mesh. As a fashion editor I quickly learned to always balance casual and formal and be on call style-wise with plenty of extras. Since we can't haul around a bag full of accessories and clothing for quick changes, here's what works for those days and situations when you never know: Always stash in your bag or tote a red lipstick, the opposite of whatever shoes you're wearing (heels or flats), and a colorful cashmere cardigan or scarf.

Combine dress up and dress down elements when you're unsure.

Here's an example: You're heading to a new neighbor get-together and have no idea how casual or dressed to get. Style down with a base of slim cropped khakis but style up with a feminine blouse and peep-toe platform pumps or metallic flats.

10. Wear the right leggings.

Black leggings are cheap and available everywhere. I half expect to see them on street corners in kiosks or vending machines any day now. Let's be honest, any leggings work for watching TV or curling up with your Kindle.

But when leggings are pressed into pants service you want the thickest, most opaque, matte black ones that you can find. They always work with knee-high boots. Don't even think about wearing them with stilettos.

Leggings should be replaced frequently since they do fade, get shiny, baggier at the seat and knees, and looser at the waist after repeated washings. One brand of leggings has stolen my heart. They're Lisse ($58, barenecessities.com), made from a thick, dense, totally opaque fabric with the kind of built-in stomach control you get from shapewear. They make ordinary generic black cotton leggings feel like plain old pantyhose. Look for thick dense ponte knit leggings too. I know, if I say ponte one more time you'll scream.

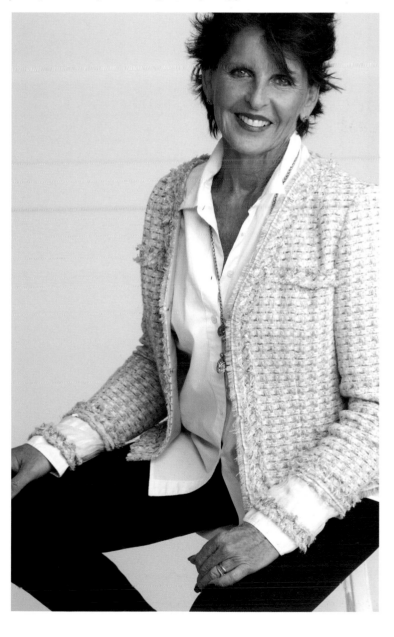

Jean Hoehn Zimmerman shows how leggings work with a Chanel jacket and a white shirt

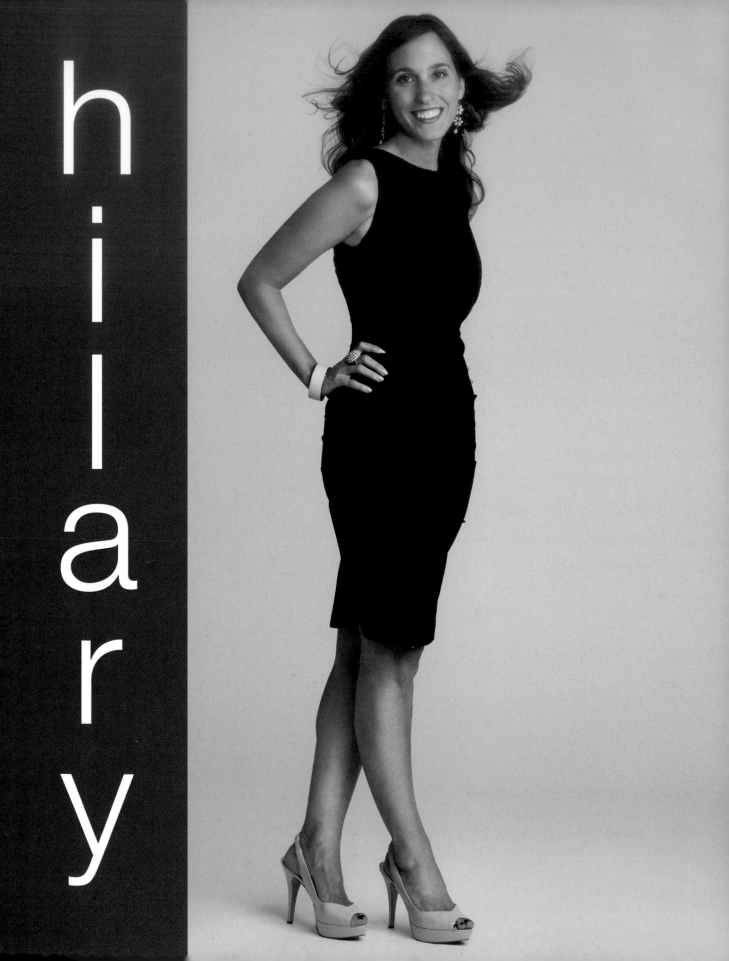

h
i
l
a
r
y

hilary on:

style: "For me it's all about marrying style with comfort. Three years ago I couldn't go anywhere without wearing three-inch heels; now I find I don't have the patience. (Thank God for wedges and riding boots!) What's changed the most is that I've begun dressing a lot more casually, although for work I find slipping on a dress is a lot less to think about."

age and fashion: "I tend not to be influenced by what my friends wear, since I'm a big believer in wearing what's most flattering, end of story. For me this means bootcut jeans, A-line dresses, and skirts and tops that emphasize my waist. I think ageless fashion is all about dressing appropriately for your body type. Most trends can be modified for any age. The key is to choose the styles that make you look fantastic."

hilary black

Executive Editor at *National Geographic*, Adult Book Division

TRADE SECRETS

EIGHT ESSENTIAL THINGS EVERY WOMAN MUST KNOW BY 40:

1. BREAK IN NEW SHOES WITHOUT KILLING YOUR FEET.

Painful shoes are like limited-edition perfumes; eventually you will tire of them or they will leave your life. If you always get blisters the first time you wear new pumps here's the preventative tip:

- **Prep the shoes** by wearing them around the house with lightweight trouser socks (not athletic or thick ones) for a week before they debut. This slightly stretches and loosens the fit. Then before the first real outing, pad the insides with inserts and gel liners at strategic points of irritation—knuckles of small toes, heels, and balls of feet. This is comparable to athletes wearing protective padding and helmets during the big game, simply part of the price to pay for wearing heels or shoes you simply can't resist.

2. LEARN TO TIE A SCARF ONCE AND FOR ALL.

These six techniques are all you need to know. Memorize and practice.

- **The French way to do a long scarf:** This is the sophisticated way to wear a long scarf. It works with long flat-knits in cashmere or wool — the kind that used to be called mufflers. Fold the scarf in half, bringing the ends together. Drape it evenly around your neck so the ends dangle in front. Slide the two loose ends through the loop and adjust the fit. This method does not give you a choked-up feeling and allows you to add a quick pop of color.

- **Fake a cowl or turtle.** This alternative technique also uses a long flat-knit scarf to extend a low-neck sweater for warmth under a coat or parka. Match the scarf to the sweater for a chic look. You can unwrap it once inside and let the ends dangle to reveal the neck and your elongating low neckline. Simply drape the scarf around your neck at the nape so the ends fall forward. Wrap the ends twice around the neck until the ends hang forward again and loop them in a loose, casual way. The degree of tautness around the neck creates a turtle or cowl effect.

- **Wrap like a rock star.** This scarf trick makes tailored jackets look edgy. It works best with dressier, long, light scarves. A simple silk menswear scarf in white or black with fringed edges is perfect, but try supple panne velvet, chiffon, and metallics too. Hold the scarf horizontally in front of your neck with the center at your Adam's apple. Cross both ends of the scarf behind your nape and bring them forward to dangle in front. Leave the ends as is or cross again if the scarf is super long.

- **Drape a big square like a jet-setter.** This scarf technique is used with an oversized silk, cotton, rayon, wool challis, or super-light cashmere square. Anything from Hermès to flea-market finds are great, especially prints. Fold the scarf in half to form a big triangle. Take hold of the points at opposite ends of the fold and cross them in back of your neck so the scarf sits in front like a bib. Then bring both ends forward to dangle or gently knot them under or over the triangle. Adjust the scarf to fall in irregular, loose folds.

• **Turn a silk scarf into a chunky statement necklace.** Fold a big silk square into an elongated shape by laying the scarf flat. Bring two opposite points in to meet at the center. Then fold in again and again until you have created a long narrow band, about an inch in width. You have two choices: Knot the scarf in the center of the band and position it in front of your neck at the hollow of your throat, where a chunky necklace would sit. Cross the ends behind your neck, bring them forward, and tie in front. The other option is to forget the knot and just center the narrow band you've created in back of your neck. Then bring the ends forward and cross them loosely around one another once and then again. Bring the ends to the back of the neck and tie in a knot. Experiment. Twisting the scarf band before wrapping makes another variation.

• **Turn a silk scarf into an evening bag.** Stretch a big silk scarf flat on your bed. In the center of the scarf place your essentials for going out. Take two opposite corners on the diagonal and tie in a knot. Take the remaining two corners and knot.

3. FAKE A SUPPORT BRA WITH A SAFETY PIN.

To get an instant lift and the effect of a minimizer bra without wearing one, simply use a big safety pin. I actually use an old-fashioned diaper pin for safety to fake a T-back or racerback bra.

Grab your bra straps together at the center of your back in an X formation and pin them together securely.

The tension lifts your boobs and eliminates sag. It also works when the armholes of a dress are deeply sculpted and you want to be sure your bra straps won't slip into view. I've used this trick thousands of times on shoots where models, celebs, and real women have shown up in the wrong bra for the wrong clothes.

4. Know how to look good behind a desk, restaurant table, or podium.

Most women know their upper body is where 99 percent of the attention goes in these situations. When you have an important meeting, lunch, dinner, or you're a featured speaker, all that counts is waist up—what I call tabletop style. Wear your hair down—not up or pulled back—and add some volume, body, and movement. This gives you an overall youthful look even when you're wearing ultra conservative clothes. Add a dazzling chunky necklace—something gutsy and almost over-the-top with fake crystals, colored stones, and lots of sparkle. We're not looking for a dainty chain or heirloom pearls here. Go for bold.

Wear a solid color dress in a vibrant or glowing color—some sort of red always exudes power, glamour, youth, and confidence in one go.

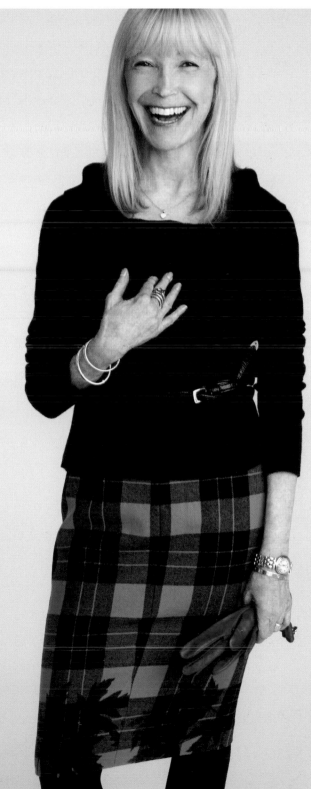

5. DO A GOOD TEMPORARY HEM.

Have you ever snagged a skirt hem getting out of the car, caught a pant hems on the heel of your shoe, or just wanted to quickly take up new jeans an inch for an evening out?

If you simply can't wait to get to the tailor (and hate ironing as I much as I do) simply tuck the fabric in place and apply a strong adhesive tape to keep it there.

Tape is preferable to pins or staples but I find ordinary office and masking tape too wimpy. Electrical tape that is stretchy and vinyl-coated or gaffer's tape (a matte finish vinyl coated cloth tape used in film studios) are sturdier and hold for the entire day or evening. They both remove without any residue. I always have rolls of these tapes around the house and in my styling kit but Hollywood Temporary Hem Tape comes in strips to make hem maintenance easy. I keep that in my car and desk.

6. MAKE A BELT WHEN YOU DON'T HAVE ONE.

Ribbons and scarves make effective stand-ins for belts. Keep a roll of thick black matte grosgrain ribbon or a black velvet tubular cord (available on ribbon and trimmings sites). Cut to triple your waist size to leave room for a generous bow. It looks feminine and sharp at the same time. Silk scarves can double as waist defining belts. Simply fold a large silky print scarf into a long, narrow shape (as in the scarf necklace technique on page 152) and knot at the waist or through the loops of your jeans.

7. TIE A SARONG, AND GET IN AND OUT OF A POOL.

Every woman needs to know how to wrap a sarong without adding excess bulk and width at the waist and hips. Badly wrapped pareos are a habit some women start making in their twenties and never change. Lose the towel!

The secret is to always start off with a non-slip cotton fabric that is soft, matte, and lightweight. The lighter the better because it is easier to drape and tie.

A print is best since it adds extra opacity and blurs bulges. Start by holding the sarong squarely behind you at waist level. Grab the top edge of the fabric on either side about twelve inches from your waist rather than at the ends. Knot these "fingers" of grabbed fabric in front at the waist or just slightly below—not at the hips. The excess ends of the fabric will be dangling. Take one dangling corner and bring it across your tummy. Tuck it into the waistband you have created. Let the other end fall free in graceful folds. This is so much better than swaddling your suit with a towel! Walk to the edge of the pool. Sit on the side, legs over the edge, and unknot the pareo just before sliding in. When you get out, grab the pareo and tie it as you exit by the stairs.

8. TURN A SWEATER INTO A LAST-MINUTE WRAP SKIRT.

I sort of learned this trick from Donna Karan. We had taken our daughters, Gabby and Jennifer, up to summer camp and were preparing to go into the lake. Donna emerged from the cabin in one of her swimsuit designs. It had two arm-like wraps that tied in front. It was a genius design and it made me think about using men's cardigans the same way.

Simply step into the cardigan at the neck (undo a few buttons first, of course). Pull the neckline up to your waist in back, button it up and tie the arms at the front to create a wrapped look.

TRADE SECRETS

g l o r i a

gloria on:

age and fashion: "I hate when magazines break up trends according to age—'Wear this in your thirties,' 'Wear this in your forties.' There are no rules. I think a fifty-year-old woman can wear what a thirty-year-old woman can wear for the most part, but she has to be more careful with beauty trends. At a certain point you make up your own rules."

wardrobe: "I wear a lot of leather jackets (especially those by Rick Owen), pants, and interesting tops. As a designer, Azzedine Alaïa works for me and my body because I have a small waist and his body-hugging, waist-defining dresses are my idea of sexy now. They're a kneeish length and feel great to wear."

real life: "We travel a lot and for some reason I am the most minimalist, efficient packer. Everything I take is black and fits in one bag—black pants, tees or sweaters, a cardigan, a black coat, two pairs of shoes, tights and tank for gym, and sunglasses. If I need something I'll buy it."

gloria appel

Former EVP at Grey Global, 30+ year career as advertising executive

I'm Obsessed with . . .

Sometimes age gets in the way of life and style. Ageless women lie about their age, marry or date men ten years younger (and talk about it), have seen *White Palace*, *How Stella Got Her Groove Back*, and *Unfaithful* with Diane Lane ten times, take Bikram yoga, drive a Mini Cooper, and wouldn't be caught dead without self-tanner. Age-appropriate women lie about their age or don't give it, divorce husbands after thirty years (quietly), have seen *Something's Gotta Give* and *It's Complicated* with Meryl Streep ten times, go to spas, drive a Benz, and wouldn't be caught dead without a bra.

If you're stuck on:

Dressing like you always have. It's time to get realistic. Unless you had an amazing facelift and are a total gym junkie I don't think you can or should look exactly the same. What you can do is maintain your overall style but keep tweaking it to stay modern. If you've always worn jeans or tailored clothes, no reason to stop now; just keep the silhouette slim and close to the body, show some skin at the neck, get a casually layered haircut, and always wear new shoes to keep the look right now.

Pulling together a great look every day. Keep it simple. Who needs to make decisions at 7 a.m.? Find your "uniform." Dress and shoes are all it takes for the office. They give your wardrobe core stability but allow you to add lots of extras fast. Change your bag no more than once a week if not once a season. Otherwise rely on your choice of jeans or leggings and layer up.

Getting Older!

Still wearing minis. Make those years of self-assurance, experience, and common sense work for you now. Would it kill you to take it down an inch or two? If you have the most incredible legs, think about how short you can go without looking stuck in a time warp. Best places to risk a mini: beachside at a resort, with tights, long layers, and tall boots in winter.

Looking up to date. Your clothes, brain, and attitude need to be on the same page. After 40 wearing the trendiest designer clothes in the world won't matter if all you can talk about is fashion and gossip. Brains and style are what really make women attractive now. Check out women TV anchors and talk show hosts like Hoda Kotb and Kathie Lee Gifford, Gayle King, Katie Couric, and Rosanna Scotto. They always wear stylish contemporary clothes but talk up a storm about life, politics, issues, personalities, world events, and news in an informed, opinionated way. You never notice the clothes except in a good way . . . second.

The Age and Fashion Mistakes Women Make

If your body took out a personal ad, here's what it would say: "Loves Shoes. Needs Clothes. Wanted: reasons to splurge and a flattery-back guarantee. Age not a problem. Age-appropriate not an issue unless you make it one."

LET'S ALL NOT:

Get too girly. I know how feminine and flattering the color pink can be. After all don't we dab a little pink cream blush high on our cheekbones for zing? But add pink to bows, puffy sleeves, ruffles, florals, dots, and sparkle and you get a major unflat-tering sugar rush. Three changes allow you to keep the color, lose the sweetness.

1) Choose nude shades of pink, apricot-pink, or rose instead of bubble gum or ballerina shades.

2) Wear pink in serious tailored clothes—knife pleat skirts, pencils, jackets, and dress pants.

3) Wear pink with black, gray, nude, or ivory.

Try to look like a model in a fashion magazine. Models are an entirely different breed; aside from the age factor, their extended body pro-portions and bone structure were not achievable when we were 20, so why would they be now?

Try to look rich. Here's what really looks luxurious: impeccable grooming. Maintenance and great shoes say money more than anything else. If you want to look like a billionaire film director, Internet mogul, or tycoon, keep your roots touched up, your body in shape, your nails and skin flawless, your teeth white and gleaming—and then add the best shoes.

Wear clunky, trendy shoes. Crazy fashion-y clodhoppers with huge chunky soles, six-inch heels and platforms, a big super-extreme shape, and snub toe shoes do not help your legs, your body, or your overall style. By next season you and your feet will wish you hadn't.

Peggy Northrop in a chartreuse coat that makes a statement

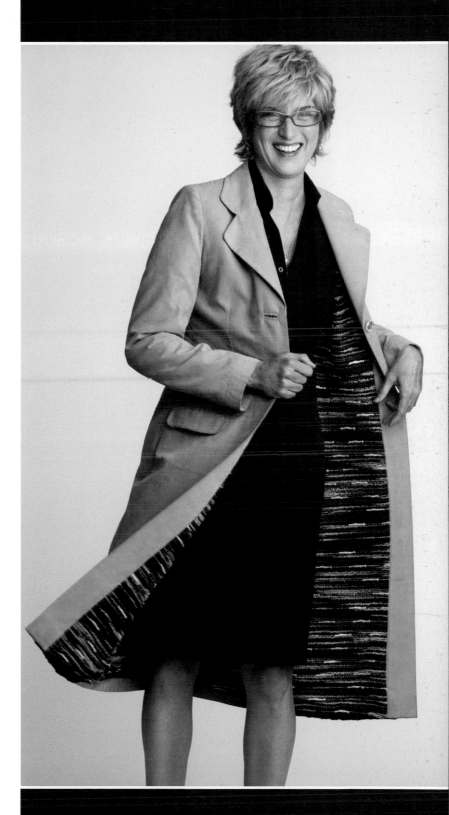

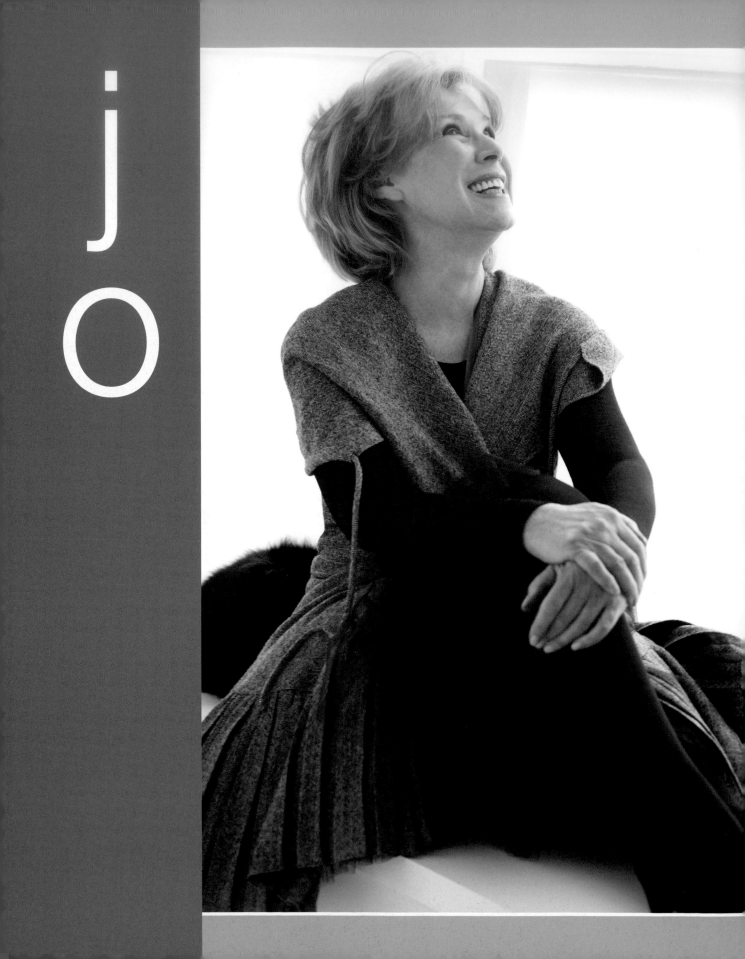

jo

jo on:

inspiration:
"Style is who you are, not what you wear. Posture is very important and I have my mother to thank for that. Holding your head high, and keeping your core centered and strong creates an aura of good carriage and poise that helps you wear clothes well."

age and fashion:
"If you're beautiful at 16, you're beautiful at 30, 50, and 70, just different. I like to twinkle, look feminine, and have dignity. I wear my star earrings to remind myself of that. They are a gift from my husband Gordon, who truly gets me. Recently I've gotten back into wearing three-inch heels after a break from them. It's one of the payoffs of exercise. I love high platform wedges too. They're feminine and easy to walk in. Sleeveless is my peeve. I've never had great arms; shrugs are terrific for solving that issue."

jo gaynor
Board member of Stephen Gaynor School, multimedia creator

CHAPTER FIVE

TO WORK OR NOT TO WORK . . .

Like it or not, it's a younger working world. Address your "packaging" or look out of touch!

Whether you are going back to work, switching careers, moving on after a reorganization, a downsizing, or plain old job loss, expect a lot of fashion changes. The way women

Felicia Milewicz

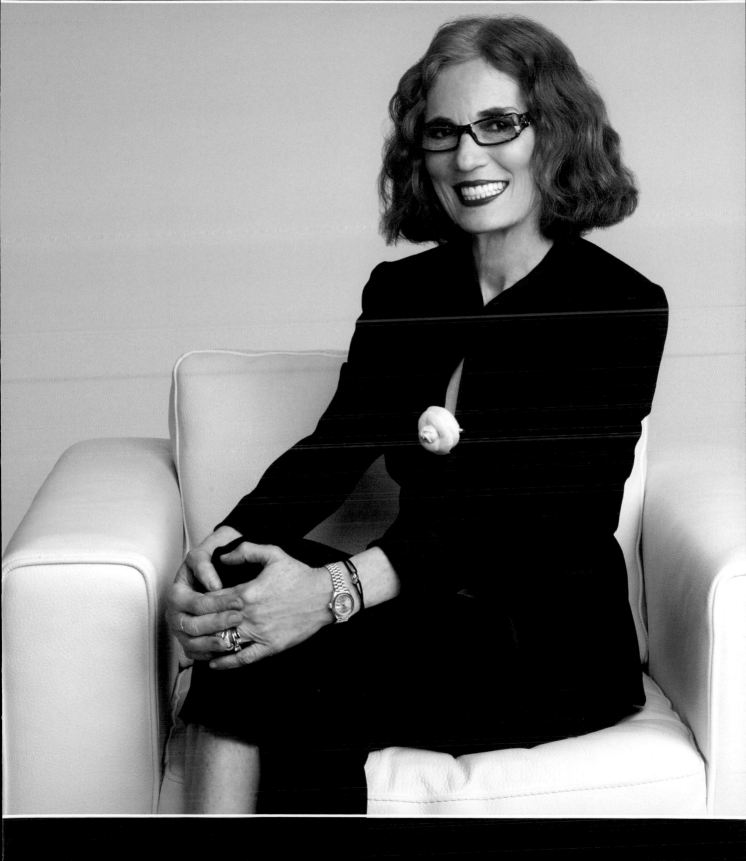

dress for work now has been impacted by major sociological shifts and technology. It doesn't matter what you do or where you work. Everyone from lawyers to financial planners to high school teachers and marketing managers are dressing more creatively.

Fashion is, after all, an instant form of communication. How you dress for work reveals a lot about your self-esteem, your attitude towards life and your body and respect for the job you perform. Recruiters, headhunters, and HR directors tally all of this when considering candidates. You only have a few minutes at the initial interview to make an impact. After you're hired you need to maintain the impression that got you there.

Here's the real backstory

If you're over 40, people you work with now may or may not know (or care) that you had a long, successful career. It's very possible to find yourself in a totally new work environment with your past really behind you.

- **You may be sitting in a cube all day and not going to meetings or presentations anymore.** Cubicles are *the* social drop-in spots. They're where you learn inside info and scoop from colleagues. Window-shop online when no one's around, listen to gossip from your chatty younger co-workers but don't add or pass any along yourself.

- **You may have taken a job that starts at 9 a.m. and ends at 5 p.m. sharp.** Maybe there's no need to check e-mails and voice-mail 24/7 like you did in your old job. Think of this as a bonus—you finally get to shape up at the gym or go for a run after work.

- **You may be telecommuting, working in a satellite office, or from home.** Your extensive work wardrobe may now feel superfluous. Rethink and remix the pieces before you toss. Your screen image still needs to be businesslike.

- **You might be a freelancer working with a new team of colleagues every couple of weeks.** Great, you can actually buy less, but buy better, or wear the same things over and over!

- **You may be temping or doing low-level office work.** Maybe you're answering phones or making photocopies. Get up to speed on technology and use the opportunity to network and job hunt. Dress up for the job you want, not the one you currently have.

- **You may be starting your own business or consulting.** You need executive polish now more than ever. Chic it up.

- **You might be doing volunteer work or fundraising to network and get your résumé around.** Even dressed down you need to show your full potential. Stay polished and groomed.

Gloria Appel in Prada
dress and gladiators

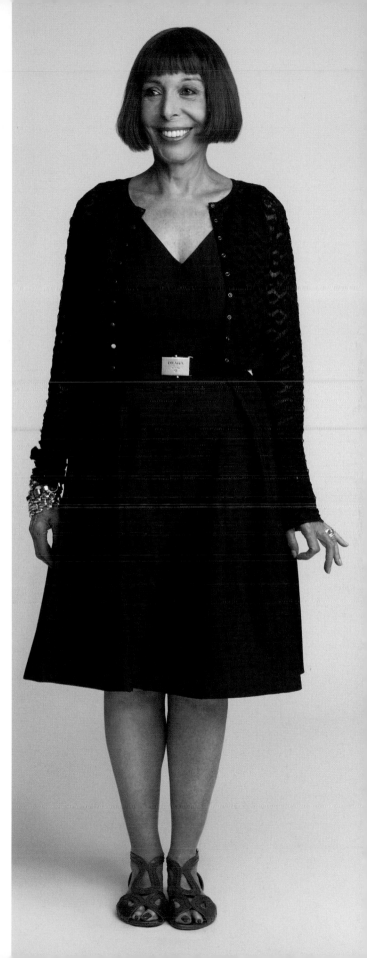

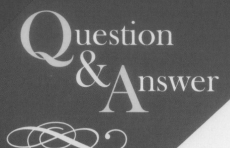

Question & Answer

Q: When your colleagues, boss, or senior manager are your daughter's age, should you trend up?

A: Updated clothes and polished style wrap your skills and abilities in a modern package—staying current keeps you in the game.

"My job left me for a younger woman" is a not-so-funny phrase making the rounds these days as more women in their forties, fifties, and sixties suddenly find themselves out of work and job hunting. It's not easy to get a grip on what to wear. We want to be seen as experienced but up to date even if we've been out of work for a few years. Some of us are taking a U-turn with lower-paying jobs that offer a chance to learn new skills, use our knowledge in a fresh way, or just get a cash flow going again.

What a wardrobe work-over does for you now

Rethink your clothes, get over your past, and dress for now. Whether you're in a job, looking for one, or working a whole new way, your clothes are part of the game. If you're still interviewing, the goal is to sell yourself past your age, beyond your experience and class-A résumé.

Me too! Same thing!

Ten years into my job as a founding editor and beauty and fashion director of *MORE* magazine I suddenly found myself going freelance. My first instinct was to look for a similar full-time gig at another magazine. Then the new-to-me world of Internet publishing and book deals beckoned. I was intrigued by the idea of working from home but bummed out about the dressed-down lifestyle that loomed ahead. Eventually I got into a new rhythm and jeans. Working "invisibly" at my computer each day with only Louie my Yorkie-Poo as "staff," I still wear makeup, jewelry, and accessories. It gives my day a sense of structure and discipline. When commuting to the city for meetings and business lunches once a week I really do dress up—more than when I was heading a dual editorial department and working with the same people every day.

My clients are all in the beauty, fashion, and publishing business so personal style plays a big role in my presentation. Some know my work but others know me only by reputation. It's essential to look fashionable and newsy all the time. I'm usually scrambling for a salon blow-out, a root refresher, and a manicure the day before these meetings . . . just like you.

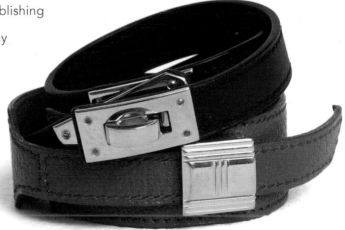

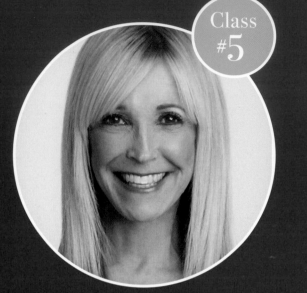

Class #5

10 Tips on Dressing for Work When Everything's Changed!

We want to look relevant and ready to go. Lots of us are now working with much younger women who wear work clothes in a new, hip way or in workplaces where the code is strictly dress-down casual. Pay attention, there's a lot to be learned there.

1. Wow them at the interview.

A job interview is a first date. What you wear matters more than ever. With fierce competition for jobs and serious unemployment problems for women 40+, our impressive résumés are unfortunately not always enough to open doors. Even women with twenty to thirty years of career-building have edited down their résumés to show only the last ten years. What you've done lately is all that really seems to matter. How you look and dress right this minute is what counts too. Keep in mind your interviewer will probably be younger than you are and dress in a contemporary (non-corporate) way no matter what the industry or job. Trust me on this one. You don't want to upstage them with a severely grown-up look, remind them of their mother, or dress down in an attempt to look youthful.

If you're interviewing for a serious corporate workplace or traditional company:

Get something new to wear. Keep it tailored, updated, and be groomed to death. If you're searching your closet for an interview outfit, skip old designer suits. No matter how much they cost back in the day or scream rich, money, power, you need to look contemporary. You may have only one chance to get it right.

Make your first choice a dress. Stick to a structured knee-length dress with or without a complementary jacket or coat (depending on the climate, season, and workplace), your first choice. It looks modern and projects confidence.

Second choice is a suit. Second choice for an initial interview would be a skirt suit but not a stuffy traditional one. Be sure it has a updated spin, like a cropped, belted, contoured, or wrapped jacket. If you never wear skirts

Peggy Northrop in yellow power/ interview dress

anymore or simply prefer pants, opt for a pantsuit but keep the shape fitted and the pants slim. You're not a rookie so don't go for a cookie-cutter dress-for-success template.

Think about color. Black, gray, or navy are always safe, assertive picks. On the other hand softer neutrals like sand, ivory, or camel can warm up your skin, make it glow, and soften expression lines and shadows under your eyes. They're a great choice when you're feeling tired, looking stressed, jet-lagged or just need a kick-in-the-pants morale boost.

Wear more color or a print for call backs. For follow-up interviews wear more color or a subtle print. It makes you memorable in the lineup of candidates who were called back. You might choose a dress in a soft coral or amber, or slip a bright print silk blouse under a jacket. How much to spend depends on your finances. When you're after a six-figure salary and a corner office you need to dress the part.

Spend on new shoes and a bag. If you're intent on nabbing the job there is one thing you must do: splurge on a better-than-average bag and classic pumps for credibility. As crazy as it sounds, HR people and recruiters check these out the minute you walk in the door. Each one I interviewed admitted to this quirk, although none agreed to be quoted. Keep nails short and manicured in a nude color, makeup fresh and natural but clearly there.

If you're up for a position in a creative industry or a "cool" job where the dress code is more casual:

Wear a newsy dress. Loosen up. Communicate your abilities but use what you wear to show your out-of-the-box thinking and personality. This is especially important if the job is in fashion, entertainment, retail, public relations, and the art or music world. A dress is going to still be a first choice here, but you have more flexibility to use color, prints, and accessories. A lot depends on the position and where the job is.

Tailored color and prints for big cities. In a formal big city like NYC, Chicago, or Dallas, make tailored sheaths, shifts, and A-lines your core interview look. Always go for color and prints instead of lost-in-the-crowd neutrals. A dress adapts quickly to changes in accessories. At the high end check out labels like Erdem, Etro, Carolina Herrera, Oscar de la Renta, Michael Kors, Donna Karan, and Akris. At the moderate end look for Diane von Furstenberg, Tory Burch, David Meister, Milly, Kay Unger, Rachel Roy, and Ann Taylor.

Add low-key trendy accessories everywhere else. If you're interviewing in a less urban or rural workplace or a city job with an informal dress code, still wear a dress for the interview. Do some research first about the company to figure out how far to take the look.

You don't want to show up in a tailored dress, ladylike bag, and serious pumps when everyone is wearing pants, jeans, and layers. Either choose a jersey dress with less structure or deconstruct a tailored dress by adding a cardigan, softer bag, and lower heel.

Do polished separates in casual workplaces. Second choice would be a non-suit look of polished separates. Choose slim pants or a tailored skirt as a base, add a blouse or fitted top, and contemporary accessories. No jeans, minis, or leggings, even if that's the overall look of employees at work and on the job.

2. When a suit is required (and sometimes it just is), get creative.

I know it's boring but suits are still expected in the legal and financial world and senior positions in many corporate offices. It doesn't matter if you're the CFO or a temp, the one thing you want to avoid is anything boring, fussy, or too traditional.

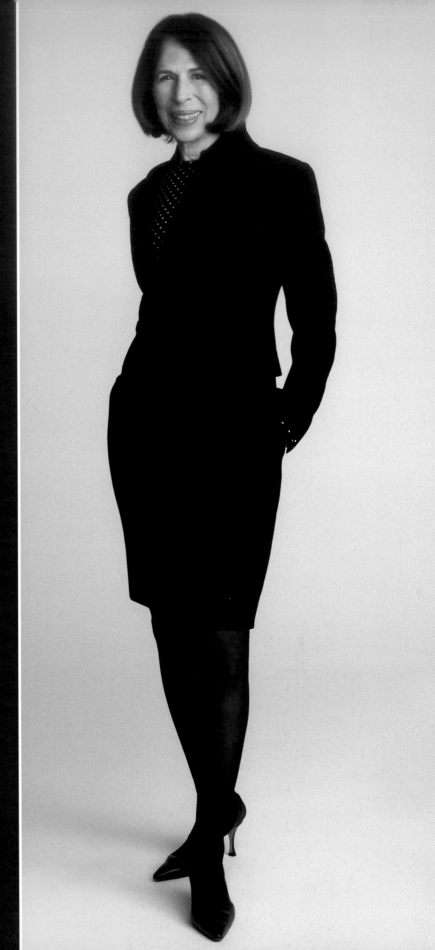

Marilyn Glass

Get an updated pantsuit.

Don't avoid pantsuits as an everyday solution even when they aren't trendy. They always remain a staple in the collections of Giorgio Armani, Ralph Lauren, and Yves Saint Laurent. If you're buying a new pantsuit choose black, with a slim tailored fit, in "lite" stretch wool or rayon, ankle cropped pants, and a cropped or hip-length jacket with a nipped waist.

3. Look for feminine jackets now.

Cardigans provide youthful, fashionable arm coverage but jackets still add a quick shot of authority. This time around don't go the same old notch collared blazer route. That's what twenty- and thirty-somethings buy when they need to look more professional and capable. We already have that going for us.

You can go for a long fitted look or a short cropped style. A long fitted jacket that is draped or cutaway at the front to reveal a slim tailored skirt beneath is one option.

Buy jackets in womanly shapes, with high armholes, slim sleeves, and feminine details. In other words, nothing that resembles a man's tailored jacket.

Stretch fabrics help contour the fit to your body and work with or without a belt. Cropped ladylike jackets are not boxy anymore and have newly slimmed down proportions. Many have ¾ sleeves, stand collars, or collarless jewel necks or wide portrait collars to show off our favorite statement necklaces and bracelets. Jackets usually last longer than bottoms when it comes to wardrobe lifespan.

4. Deal with the weather issue.

When you're young, arriving at meetings or the office soggy, soaked, and water-logged is part of the learning curve. After 40, anticipating inclement weather and preparing for it is smart style strategy. Back in the day we'd pull on sporty rain boots and change when we got to the office or wore black patent pumps that were more resistant to water and stains than our good leather shoes. Now there's a better plan.

Get slim waterproof boots. Get yourself a pair of chic, knee-high black rubber boots and a pair of waterproof stretch leather or stretch suede boots in black or brown. They look exactly like their normal polished everyday sisters but resist puddles, ice, snow drifts, and downpours. The rubber versions allow you to charge straight into a storm. They come in flat riding boot styles and fashionable chunky heels or wedges from Burberry, Hunter, Kate Spade, Jimmy Choo, Loeffler Randall, and Marc by Marc Jacobs. The waterproof stretch leather and suedes also come in flats, heels, and wedges and a huge range of ankle cropped booties or slim knee-high boots. Aquatalia by Marvin K. and La Canadienne do them but my all-time world-class favorites are by Stuart Weitzman.

Add a water-resistant coat. A knee-length down puffer with a hood or convertible large shawl collar works for cold weather; your trench for everything else. The down coat should be a neutral, shaped to fit.

Count on a stylish waterproof tote. Last, get a waterproof open top rubber tote toned to your boots for stashing your foldable umbrella, good heels, and flats. The Hunter Shopper is ideal (same brand that makes the rubber boots). You're now ready for anything.

5. Make tailored coats part of a look.

Think of tailored coats as part of an outfit rather than a last-minute add-on. Remember Michelle Obama's pre-inauguration camel coat and matching pencil skirt duo by Narciso Rodriguez? How about her green coat and dress look by Isabel Toledo at the inauguration? Or the black coat and full skirt by Jason Wu she wore to meet the queen? Suddenly a wardrobe of ladylike coats makes a huge amount of sense for working women our age. Choose light wool blends, wool crepe, cotton gabardine, and twills that don't add a lot of bulk. Be sure the separates or dress have enough professional elegance to get by solo once you remove the coat.

> Matching a light tailored coat toned to your skirt, dress, or pants provides polish without the need for a jacket.

Coats in simple, single-breasted styles look good open or closed and flatter everyone. Straight topcoats with a classic fit or A-line princess styles are first choice. Belted coats work if your waist is great. Women with hourglass figures, a small top and fuller shape below, or those with tall athletic bodies can wear a belted coat.

6. Drape and shape pencils for confidence.

Pencil skirts in all their variations are the most useful skirts to own for work. The body-skimming waist to knees shape provides a trim base whether you're a size 4 or 14. Some pencils have a fluted or fishtail flip at the hem which adds little more ease of movement—great if you have full thighs. Pencils with subtle draping disguise weight issues, stomach bloat, and bulges and are comfortable to wear.

These three tailored skirts provide the best solutions:

A draped pencil sits low on the waist but has no waistband. It's smooth across the rear but gathers across the tummy in a graceful fold like a sarong.

A tulip-shaped pencil has vertical tucks at the waist (like a starburst) to ease the fabric gently over the tummy before tapering towards the hem.

A faux-wrap pencil has an extra layer of fabric across the stomach but keeps the slim pencil shape.

Choose supple fabrics like viscose, polyester, and wool blends that drape well and add elongating, tapered-toe shoes with some sort of heel to balance the subtle extra fullness across the stomach and hip area.

7. Don't get too casual, even if everyone else does.

What looks fashionably relaxed on a twenty or thirty-year-old in a dress-casual work environment can look sloppy when you're 40, 50, and 60. If the dress code is so relaxed that everyone wears jeans or leggings, stick to jeans or jersey dresses. Choose your favorite jean fit relaxed or tight in a dark, even wash and layer up on top in serious neutrals (see Chapter 1 for how-tos) or add a tailored jacket for extra polish. Add personality with scarves, jewelry, distinctive reading glasses, and belts—and of course great shoes or boots.

Dresses in soft jerseys and knits are relaxed yet professional. The shoes and bags you choose can push the look further in either direction.

Any item of clothing that reveals your back, chest, feet, stomach, or underwear is not okay for work. No sundresses, sweats, shorts, or flip-flops. No scrunchies, leggings, message tees, sequins, lamé, or glitter polish. Younger staffers may get away with it in the most dressed-down workplaces; we simply can't—even if you're working at a five-star beach resort or on a college campus.

8. Get your fashion fix with shoes.

Work shoes always need updating. Play with heel height but don't fool around with other color and style options unless you have nude and black covered.

Three work basics are crucial: skin-tone nude pumps, classy black heels, and sleek, tapered, neutral flats.

If you have to choose, upgrade the quality of your basic nude and black work shoes before updating the look with trendier details. Then move on to updating texture—adding embossed croc, snakeskin, and patent leather to your basic nude and black leather. Third, add leopard heels before moving on to color. In a classic pump these work like a neutral and de-stuff any tailored outfit in less than sixty seconds. Stacked heels and D'Orsay pumps with cutouts at the instep balance curvy calves and heavy ankles. They also flatter legs that tend to get puffier below the ankles as the day progresses. Refined, ladylike heels in T-strap and Mary Jane styles are good options for feet that have lost padding and support with age. Unless you're a masochist or work at a fashion magazine, chances are you're not running around in six-inch-platform heels everyday, but foldable ballet flats slip into any bag and are a smart idea for everyone. Check out those from Gap and CitySlips. They make work commutes, driving, and the allover to and fro ing of daily work life easy.

9. Keep updating your glasses.

Even if you usually wear contacts there will be days when you can't. Put getting new-looking glasses on your to-do list. This is not a one-shot deal. Eyeglasses change slightly every couple of years in size, shape, and color so updates every year or two make a difference. The last thing you want to wear at work are aging eyeglasses.

Cool, modern glasses are essentially face jewelry. They frame your eyes, drive attention to the upper face (and away from your neck and jaw line), and hide squint lines.

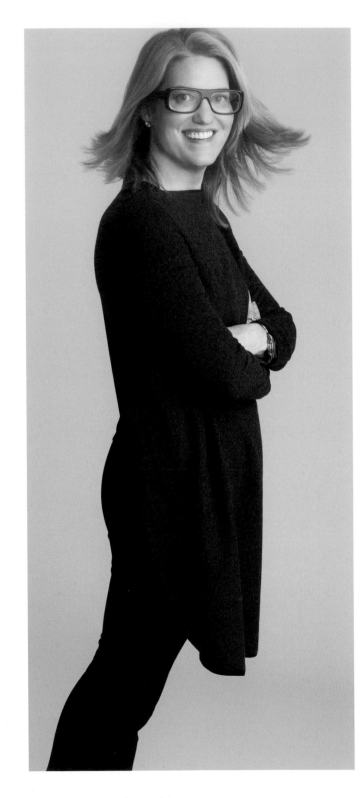

Right now the trend is towards strong black or tortoiseshell frames with a squared, masculine look or big strong cat-eye shaped frames. Both styles work like emphatic eye-liner to add extra definition to your face and a subtle sexiness to serious work clothes. My own work glasses are bold black frames by Cutler and Gross and Tom Ford—one square, the other a cat eye. Check sites like eyebobs.com, warbyparker.com, and eyefly.com for distinctive picks.

Just a reminder: the skin around your eyes is thin, dry, and prone to wrinkling and puffiness. It's the give-away zone for age, stress, insomnia, and work overload. Be strategic; glasses can hide a lot. Slightly tinted lenses can make circles less obvious and a subtle cat eye frame can lift saggy lids and minimize the elevens (the vertical creases between your brows).

Jane Larkworthy in cool glasses, tunic, and slim black pants

10. Get into camel
pants, dress, and skirt ASAP.

This color happens to work for every skin tone and adds a golden sun-warmed, healthy glow to mature skin.

Camel is magical on us and it's surprisingly the most underrated, under-explored neutral for work. If you're used to buying tailored work pieces in dark, cool colors you're in for a shock. Wear camel pieces head-to-toe or mix them tonally. It looks drop-dead chic with black but also teams up with chocolate, gray, red, ivory, and leopard. Start out with a few central basics and then add a camel coat, tees, and sweaters. This super-flattering hue is getting a lot easier to find year-round now that "nude" shades have become an expanded fashion color theme; Michael Kors and J.Crew are always reliable sources.

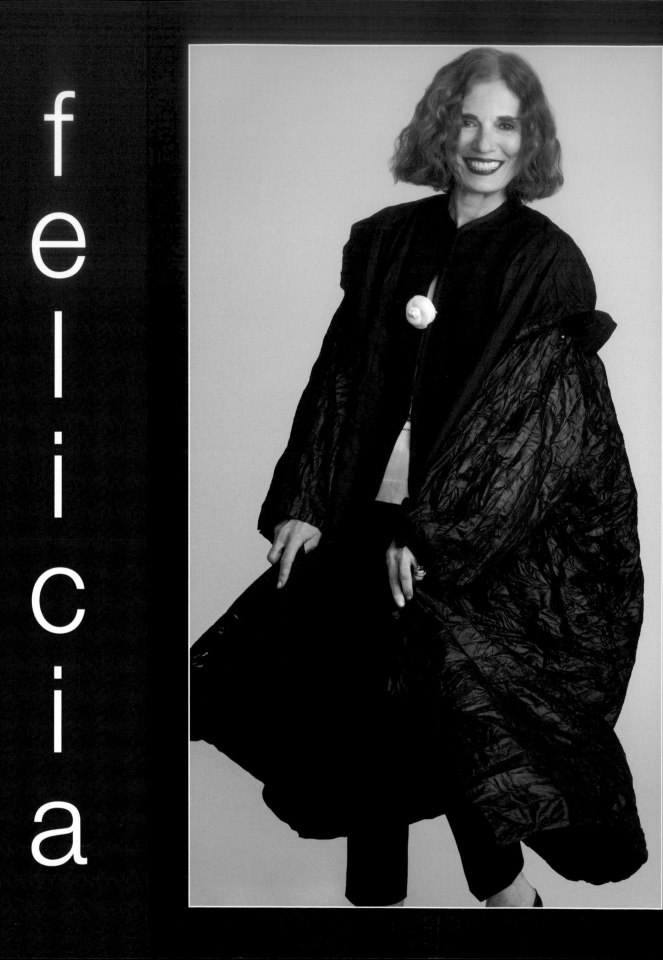

felicia

felicia on:

style: "For me comfort is #1. I don't look for trends although a touch is always great if it works out that way. One thing I do is never plan what to wear in advance. Whether it's an event or just getting dressed for work in the morning I make that decision in the moment. Lately, I live in pants and like to mismatch suits."

wardrobe: "I don't wear color—only black or white. What I don't wear I give away to charity. I mostly wear pants, Chanel ballet slippers, sweaters, blouses, and tailored jackets. I save beautiful old suits by getting them retailored. The only kind of jewelry I wear is personal—something with meaning like my gold Rolex, my wedding ring, and pearls. I love good bags but I stick to one a season and I prefer those not too large or heavy."

felicia milewicz
Beauty Director, *Glamour* magazine

TRADE SECRETS

PARE IT DOWN OR LAYER UP.

When your boss or manager is twenty years younger than you are:
Freshly whitened teeth and a dark edgy nail color go a long way towards fitting in. That done, update your clothes one of two ways. Either go minimalist with a one-color theme or layer your clothes up for a hipper feeling. Here's an example: you might pair navy pants with a navy sweater or navy shirt for a sleek Jil Sander/Calvin Klein minimalist look or cinch them with a brown croc belt, over layers of tanks and tees, and top it off with a slouchy gray cashmere cardigan.

WEAR FRIENDLY COLORS AND APPROACHABLE PRINTS.

When you want your co-workers and boss to see you as a team player: Let your clothes reflect that attitude. Wear something upbeat in red, yellow, or orange for meetings, business lunches, workshops, and when asking for a raise or promotion. This cheery palette includes sophisticated, trendy, or classic shades like coral, hot pink, tomato, acid-yellow, or raspberry. Add shine near your face too—anything from big gold hoops to a rosy-pink lip gloss looks welcoming. I think of this as "say-yes-dressing."

Jean Hoehn Zimmerman in feminine jacket, belted, with ties at wrists over a tailored base. Friendly, energetic red peps up black and white.

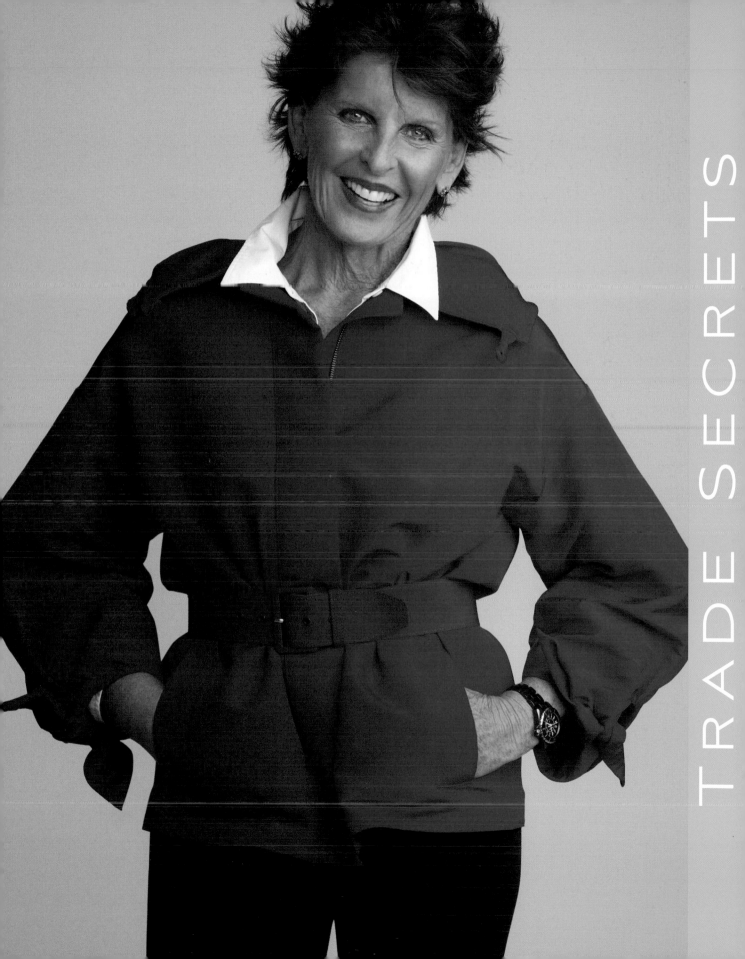

Break down an ultra-conservative look.

When you don't want to look too traditional in classic suits, blazers, tweeds, and pinstripes: Haul them in to the tailor. Then all you need are belts to shape the jackets and add attitude, knit V-neck sweaters to match all your pants and skirts, and a slightly trendier shoe. All give very businesslike pieces a more feminine, contemporary look. Fashion is a big game—if you have solid core pieces and a few extras you can't go wrong. Just be sure to update the shoes.

Improvise a business look without wearing a suit.

When you vowed never to wear suits again and your new office is corporate or conservative and suits are the usual attire: Fake it. Structured knee-length dresses in neutrals, pinstripes, or tweed worn with quality pumps, a good bag, and non-jangly jewelry will look correct. For meetings throw on a toned-to-match jacket and belt it over the dress or select a cropped jacket for polish. The look will read as a three-piece skirted suit. Don't try to sneak in knits or soft jersey dresses, but a tailored peplum top and trim skirt can work too.

Take the drag out of a new commute to work.

When you have a long daily commute or the suburban to urban trek is breaking your fashion spirit: Rethink your travel gear. First of all there's the weather, then the big drag of carrying your laptop, workbag, coffee, and your usual handbag, and finally the reality of standing/sitting for extended periods of time. Wear flats during the commute and change your shoes upon arrival.

Stick to ankle cropped pants and skirts or dresses rather than longer pants to make the transition easy. Wear big dark glasses if you want to avoid early a.m. conversations and have your iPod for privacy.

DRESS TO SKYPE.

When you have Skype meetings or even job interviews with people in other states and countries without leaving home or your office: Look as professional and well dressed on screen as you would in person. Stick to solids—prints and patterns can be distracting. Dress at least from the waist up as if you're in a real office situation. I like to wear heels and something tailored since it improves my posture and keeps my silhouette and voice crisp. Practice in a mirror to get comfortable. Color looks assertive and energizing on screen and can help separate you from the background.

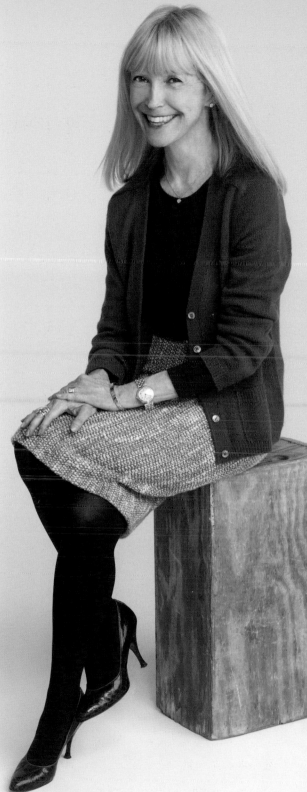

TRADE SECRETS

I'm Obsessed with . . .

Fitting in at a mostly very young workplace.

Everyone will focus 90 percent of their attention on your shoes, bag, and jewelry so don't worry too much about the clothes. Depending on the vibe—dresses, jeans, and slim pants will get you through.

Not looking like somebody's mother.

Keep surprising them with edgy touches of leather. A black leather fitted vest under a jacket, a leather pencil, or a leather jacket over a dress with boots, does it. Instead of polite florals, wear artsy prints with an abstract/graffiti/techno feel.

Whether to wear sheer hose or go barelegged.

Take cues from higher-ups. Sheer pantyhose are still a requisite in corporate offices and some industries. If the most influential staffers wear sheers so should you. However, go for

Being a Team Player But Standing Out in the Crowd.

the nudest possible and be sure skin tone matches head to toe. Nude fishnets are a good middle ground. If you self tan your legs, instead of wearing sheers remember you need to go head to toe for a uniform look.

Sneaking back to work after de-aging cosmetic surgery.

Do it over a long vacation holiday so bruising will be minimal and just look like the result of extreme travel (the long flight to Australia and back) or happy partying. Switch up your wardrobe colors. If you usually wear black, dress in white, color, or prints. Everyone will attribute the new you to that. No sunglasses indoors if you get your eyes done! Create a diversion with eye-catching jewelry. Change your hair in some way—add highlights or skip the flatiron and go for a fuller, more tousled look.

Business trips.

New frequent flyers need to know airport terminals, hotel lobbies, and meeting rooms are always freezing. Always have a huge cashmere scarf or shawl to throw on over jackets and to use as a pillow or blanket on planes. Travel in tailored, slim black pants and a jacket (your most crushable pieces) and flats. Stash a chunky necklace, low pumps, a couple of disposable toothbrushes, and another top or two in your carry-on in case you don't have time to change on arrival. Pack a chic tailored dress for meetings that glam up easily for dinner or cocktails.

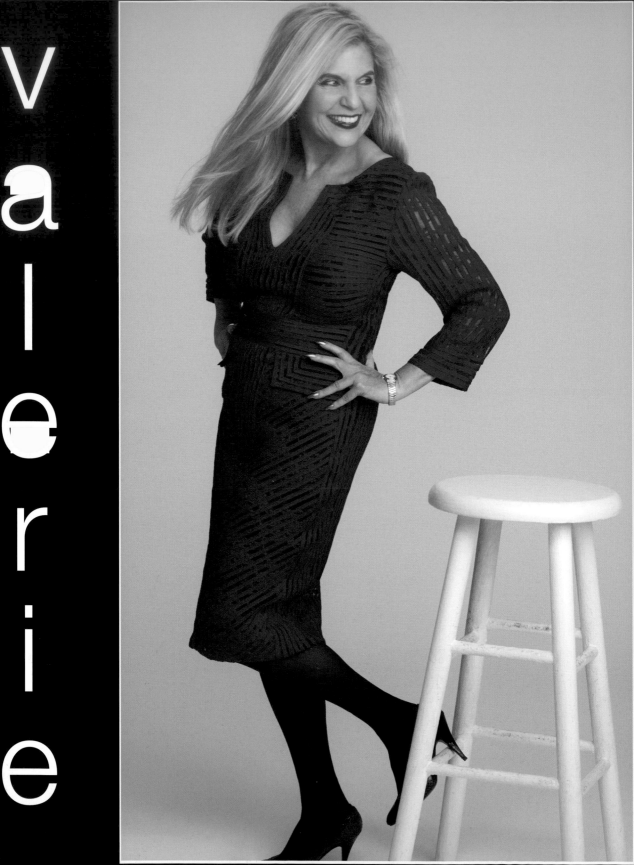

valerie

valerie on:

inspiration:
"I honestly only look through top fashion magazines like *Vogue* and *Harper's Bazaar* and high-end catalogs like Neiman Marcus to see the latest trends. Then I shop my own closet for similar looks from what I already own."

age and fashion:
"In the last two years I've gotten slimmer and have lost about 15 pounds. I'm going through a divorce and dating again so I prefer body-conscious clothes that show my assets! I'm rediscovering a lot of things I couldn't wear before, breaking up ensembles in fresh ways and actually enjoy the whole process. I don't wear minis anymore but I still like my skirts two inches above the knee. I don't wear sleeveless anymore either but a collection of shrugs makes sleeveless dresses wearable again and I do love ¾ sleeves. I no longer wear loose, full tops and I belt everything—belts make everyone look slimmer and more youthful."

current obsession:
"I have two can't-live-without items. My new gorgeous, lacey minimizer bra by Wacoal is simply the best bra I've ever owned and makes every top and dress look better. Every full-busted woman needs this bra. Next on the list is my Stuart Weitzman waterproof high-heel boots. They are indestructible in rain and snow, don't give you a clunky look, and work with dresses, knits, pants—just anything."

valerie lynn
Artist

The Work Attire Mistakes Women 40+ Make

Work clothes depend on where you work, how you work and what you do, but despite new situations some things haven't changed. A heads-up can make any transition easier. Nice thought because we're going to be working longer than men since we tend to live longer! In 2008, an estimated 62 million more women than men lived to be 65 and older. Hmmm.

LET'S ALL STOP:

Shlepping. Heavy bags carted around daily are unhealthy for us and unattractive. They cause or amplify shoulder and back strain and ruin the line of our clothes. Unfortunately, we often carry not one but several heavy bags around at once. It's fine to lug around basics but do you really need to carry that extra large water bottle, workout clothes, and snacks? Our packed, over-scheduled lifestyle encourages this mule-ish tradition and we've simply got to stop. Leave some at the office, in your car, or home.

Thinking a suit makes up for maintenance. Grooming slip-ups at work kill the most flawless track record. You might be sleeping two hours a night thanks to hot flashes or caring for

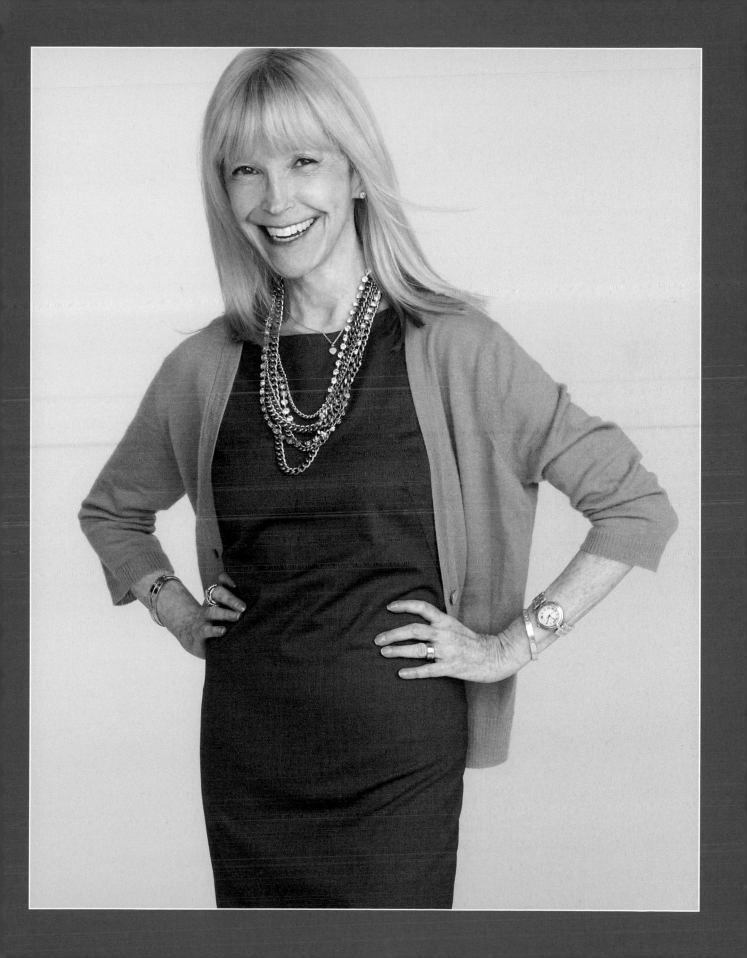

a sick parent. If it shows in your appearance look out! Scuffed shoes, run-down heels, stained clothes, lint, and/or bulges at the midriff don't make up for a great dress. Stash a lint roller in your desk and use a black permanent marker to fill in scratches and scuffs. Buff leather shoes and boots every week with a moisturizing cream. Keep your eye on the heel lift, the little strip at the bottom. Replace it when you see signs of wear, before a clicking sound signals damage.

Wearing shapewear that's too tight, bras that create bulges. Be sure shapewear is the right length for your legs and skirt. It should be short enough at the leg so you don't flash it when you sit or cross your legs. Wear camisoles and bodysuits with built-in bras to cancel out annoying bra band bulges under light blouses, knits, and dresses that your usual bra can't solve.

Playing it too safe. Certain things do work most of the time. But why would women who have made "change" their mantra play it totally safe now at work? It's time to shake

things up. Get three possible uniforms going— a dress look, a pant look, and a skirt look. Find the perfect proportions, pieces, and shapes that work for you, then swap in texture, color, and prints to add excitement.

Carrying around chic bag, crappy wallet, or dirty makeup case. Whether you're paying for lunch with a colleague, handing over a business card, or doing repairs in the ladies room, every time you pull out your wallet or makeup the cases should be clean and fresh. Look for full-size French wallets with zip around or flap closures and plenty of slots for credit cards and IDs. Choose a color you'll spot easily at the bottom of your bag. Keep make-up in a small Ziploc plastic bag and replace it every few days if a black nylon Prada one is out of the question.

Skipping makeup, thinking your clothes can do it all. According to a study released in October 2011,* wearing make-up enhances your perceived attractiveness, competence, likability, and trustworthiness in the eyes of others at work. A rosy or tawny lipstick

*Funded by Procter & Gamble and in partnership with Dana-Farber Cancer Institute and Boston University

can make you appear powerful. A tinted moisturizer, bronzing powder, or a gradual self-tanner can help you look well rested. If your
makeup looks too done or powdery under the fluorescent lighting,
dampen a makeup sponge with cold water and pat your face to remove excess foundation, blush, or bronzer, and freshen the texture.
Blend down shadow or liner, and remove under-eye smears with
a clean Q-tip.

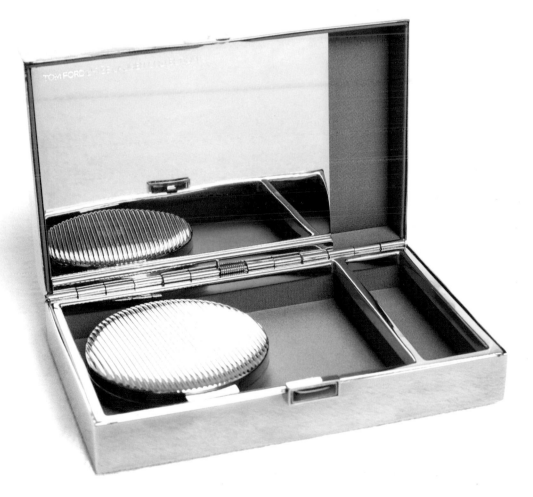

CHAPTER SIX

SO WHAT NOW?

New social and lifestyle predicaments need new solutions.

Who knew along with the perks of getting older (wisdom, experience, the ability to say no), come special fashion situations to test our true grit. You're getting married at 50? Have your first blind date in twenty years? You're the mother-of-the-bride and don't want to look like one? Pregnant (finally or again) at 45? You're retiring, moving from New York to Arizona and hate hot-weather clothes? The list of what to wear questions ramps up after 40 as new social and lifestyle predicaments accummulate.

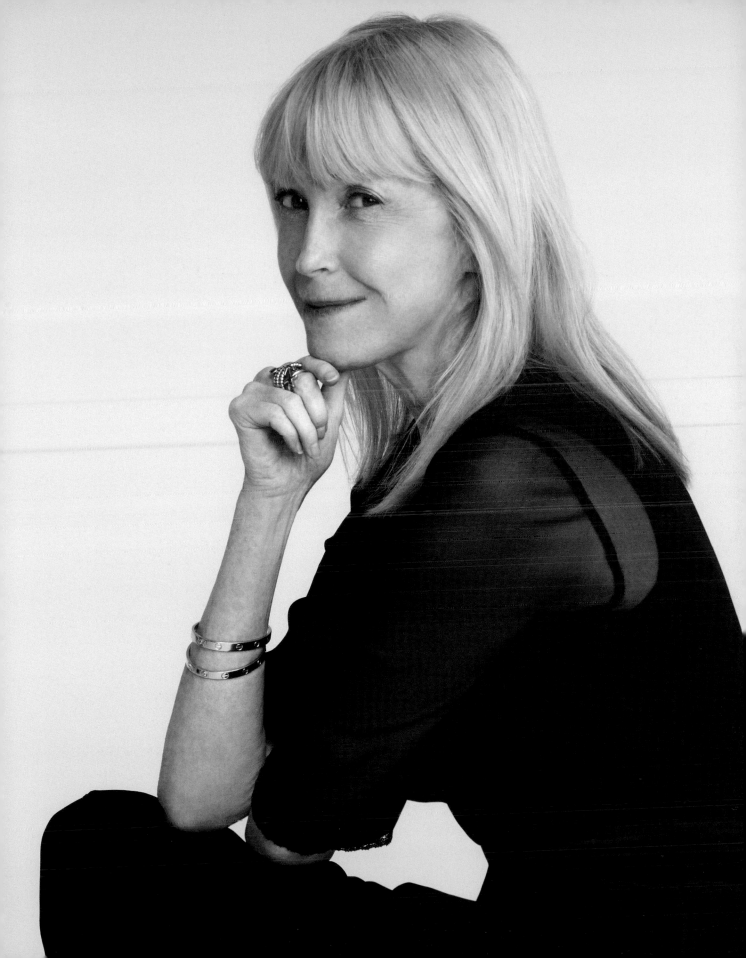

Here's the
real backstory

- **Every woman has a complicated life.** Thanks to blended families, the extension of early and mid-life situations like dating, marriage, and even pregnancy beyond 40, new opportunities, continued work years, unpredictable climate, changes in lifestyle, and social networking we have more clothes situations than ever before.

- **We travel more than ever.** We jet around to see grandkids and attend destination weddings, globe-trot for pleasure and to learn about other cultures, plan hiking trips and sightseeing vacations. We spend more time on the road in RUVs and cars and take cruises at the drop of a hat. And we're traveling for business, too! Brilliant packing strategies are essential.

- **We're dating and getting married or remarried through our seventies.** Who could have anticipated this? Social networking has re-energized our friendships, love, and sex lives.

- **We still want to do the things we love . . . and dress for them.** Rock concerts, summers at the beach, high school and college reunions make nostalgia the present.

- **We need clothes for divorce court, wakes, and memorial services.** Occasions we never thought about before have now become dress smart events.

Q: Do you think you need more clothes than ever now?

A: Nope. Just genuine real-life solutions, not some fashion fantasy.
Me too! Same thing! When my daughter Jennifer got married eleven years ago I couldn't wrap my brain around dressing as a mother-of-the-bride. Neither could she. Having grown up with a very nonconformist fashion mom, Jennifer would beg me to "please wear something normal" when I showed up for parent-teacher conferences. About a year prior to her wedding, while on a photo shoot in LA I found a perfect dress: a vintage French black couture one-shoulder gown in mint condition and my exact size at a consignment shop in Beverly Hills. It must have been purchased and never worn because the tags were still on it. I figured it would be useful to have someday and that's what I ended up wearing to her wedding. My approach to dressing for life's big moments is still the same. I buy special items right away, before I need them. Sooner or later I will. Two items I never pass up: a faux-jeweled belt or a dressy skirt. This has saved me from ever having to do last-minute event shopping . . . ever, for life.

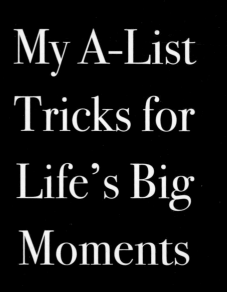

LOIS' HOTSHOT
FASHION EDITOR

Class #6

My A-List Tricks for Life's Big Moments

1. Fly like a celebrity. Look good at all times.

There's nothing like an airport for bringing out your inner slob. No one is expecting you to arrive in furs, peep-toe pumps, and a stack of Louis Vuitton trunks, but if you look a little chic you're more likely to get what you want: An up-grade, the window seat, a better room at the hotel on arrival.

No more matching velour sweat suits, super-tight jeans, flip-flops, or heels. For non-work trips stay casual but put-together.

Layer long tanks with slim ankle cropped pants, flats, and a cozy but stylish sweater you can sleep in or wear straight off the plane. Wear a hoodie or bring a pull-on knit hat plus earplugs or Bose noise-cancelling headphones so you can nap soundlessly. A long scarf is a wear or carry-on essential. I like the ease of driving shoes for the quick on-and-off but slip into warm socks on board. I prefer soft narrow cropped pants and an underwire-less bra. Legs, breasts, and feet swell during long flights so avoid the compression of items like leggings, fitted jeans, and boots. Also in your on-board bag: e-reader, medication, cell, an extra pair of undies (in case of lost or detained luggage, especially if you transfer), a moisturizer with sunscreen, and a tinted lip balm. Check almost everything. Let the new pricey pay-per-bag regulations force you to be a more efficient packer. You don't want to be a schlepper.

2. Stay a little fluid about dress codes.

Dress code definitions have changed. Don't ignore them but don't feel totally confined by the suggestions anymore. Deciding what to wear can be annoying and confusing enough without specific instructions. Do the words optional or preferred really give us wiggle room? Yes. What exactly is beach formal? Urban casual? Downtown chic?

Here's the gist of it:

White tie: Ultra formal and you do need a gown so don't try to squeeze out of wearing one.

Black tie or black tie optional: Means dress like you're going to the Oscars as a guest, not a nominee. You can certainly wear long, but a knee-length, high-neck, super glamorous dress in a luxurious fabric, and color actually gives you a lot more choice.

Cocktail party: Depends on whether it's work related, you're going straight from work, or it's a Friday or Saturday night deal where you can dress from scratch at home. After-work or work-related cocktail celebrations are where any high-neck, tailored, solid color dress really comes through for you. It adapts quickly to a change of accessories—higher or dressier heels and some statement sparkly jewelry in a necklace or earrings.

Business attire: If your workplace is relaxed and less formal, wear your most polished everyday work look. Then add one or two elements that raise the bar. A silk blouse, an embellished cardigan, a wow necklace, and a red lipstick may be all the oomph you need to transform jeans, cropped pants, or a jersey dress.

Urban casual/casual chic: For us it translates as a favorite neutral work look with a pop of color or a statement accessory. Don't overdo the shine and glitz here. You could do matched cropped pants and a slim sweater belted with a scarf and alligator cuffs, or a knit dress with python platform sandals and a stack of colorful bangles.

Beach formal: For destination weddings and celebrations when the host doesn't want guests showing up in Hawaiian shirts and sundresses. Wear a draped dress that moves and is breezy (not a sheath), and sandals since you might be barefoot part of the time. Get a pedicure!

Jean Hoehn Zimmerman in silver Oscar de la Renta evening gown: big deal wedding/event

Come as you are or casual dress: Does not mean wear your most ripped/torn/distressed jeans, tees, sweats, and sneakers . . . really. It means dress up your current favorite jeans with something that shows a little effort—like a draped top, cashmere sweater, and dressier ballet flats or boots.

3. Make one shoulder your new cleavage substitute.

Big deal evenings and super-glam parties mean go all out but not via plunging necklines, boob-revealing halters, or a strapless dress. It's all about the neckline and all three of these emphasize sag and sun damage. Your shoulders are still the one body zone you can count on practically forever to provide a crisp line. Use them as a hitching post for the dressy neckline that gives us all a sexy, strong, womanly shape and attitude: the one shoulder. Whether it's topping a knee-length dress or a floor-length gown, a one-shoulder look creates an elongated, elegant diagonal line that sleeks and slims even if you're 5'3" and a size 14.

A one-shoulder dress covers your chest yet highlights one shoulder in a deliberately sensual way that's far more flattering than showing your boobs.

4. De-stress with bodysuits and control slips.

Bodysuits should be a basic in every 40+ woman's closet. Some have skinny adjustable straps, some have wider tank straps, and some are available with ¾ or long sleeves. Certain bodysuits work as tops from the waist up and are meant to be seen. Others have extra spandex control and built-in bras and work more like extended shapewear. Both are great buys in black and white. Wolford's pricey bodysuits are really fashion pieces and the above-the-waist part looks just like a fitted silky tee. SPANX has control versions of tank bodysuits with 38 percent spandex to control flab and flatten jiggles.

The other essential is a full-body control slip to wear under dresses. Ones with a built-in bra eliminate the need for two items and are great under jersey wrap dresses and tailored knits. The SPANX Slim Cognito Shaping Full Slip, the Sassybax Pretty Slip, and the Yummie Tummie Boyfriend Slip are gorgeous yet provide a serious power surge. Stock up.

These take the stress out of getting dressed for events or just plain old everyday life.

5. Always have a backup plan. Some days you don't want to make decisions at 6 a.m. or 7 p.m. or can't deal with more than slipping on a pair of black pants. Maybe your dress didn't make it back from the dry cleaner or you suddenly can't fit into it. Sometimes dressing up is a more spontaneous thing—a dinner invitation, a date, or a last-minute party evite.

Here are the top four problems and solutions:

You're ten pounds heavier than when you bought your last dressy dress: Forget that dress for now. We usually buy dressy dresses for certain occasions after we've dieted and sweated through weeks of workouts. We then need another diet or serious shapewear to wear them again. Don't panic. Start at the bottom and create a slim base with a black pencil that actually fits and gorgeous heels. Add a neck-elongating, hip-length top in a body-skimming shape. Wear your most eye-catching statement jewelry, a memorable fragrance, and smoky lined eyes.

You had laser surgery for brown spots and can't show your chest, arms, or legs: Pull out your narrow dressy pants and add a long sleeve tunic, super fancy long sleeve blouse, or a luxurious shirt in heavy silk or lined lace. Wear a major cascade necklace or a supple embellished scarf to hide any visible redness at the upper chest.

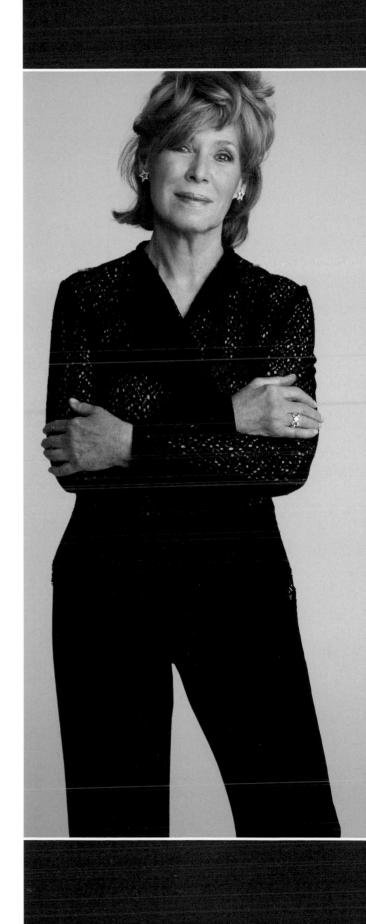

Jo Gaynor in black lace top and black pants: business dinner, last-minute dress up

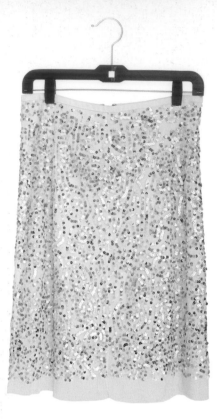

You just found out your ex/boss/crush is going to be there: Not to worry. Stretch your neck and legs of course and wear those heels! A body-skimming dress in a color that makes your skin/hair/eyes glow is more important than an impressive designer label. Don't go immediately to black (everyone will be in black). Accent your waist, wrists, collarbone, legs, or ears with a standout accessory that gleams and shines.

You forgot it was tonight: Add any sequined, velvet, or lace top to everyday tailored pants or skirts. Add any sequined, lace, or velvet pencil skirt to any solid black or white shirt or fitted top. Sequins, lace, and velvet make quick changes almost too easy. Pick up classic pieces in these dressy fabrics when you spot them on sale. Then choose one at a time. Always have two fresh pairs of sheer black pantyhose (in case you run the first in your rush to dress) and a black opaque bra and bodysuit on standby too.

6. Arm yourself
with an emergency kit.

I keep a bag of panic preventers in my closet and since I often commute to work and travel a lot, a duplicate goes in my tote or suitcase. Some of these items and a few others also go in my clutch for evening or my tote on important days.

Here are my seven saviors:

1. **Hollywood Fashion Tape** is hypoallergenic double-stick tape safe for skin and delicate fabrics to secure deep necklines and close gaps between buttons on shirts and blouses.

2. **Gal Pal Garment Deodorant Removers** are reusable dry pink sponges that get rid of deodorant, powder, and makeup but especially that annoying underarm white residue. I carry one in my bag when I wear sleeveless dresses, especially LBDs, for touchups.

3. **Tide to Go Instant Stain Remover Pen** to remove last minute spills and splotches from tea or coffee.

4. **Foot Petals** are shoe-toned cushions in a variety of innovative, feminine shapes for heels, balls of feet, and arches. They sooth and prevent blisters and calluses. They're actually great looking, so even if you slip your shoes off, the pads look like part of the shoe. They even work with bare sandals. The Foot Petals Stiletto Stylist Kit has a mix of all, but I depend on the Tip Toes (both available on footpetals.com) for ball-of-foot cushioning in slingbacks and boots.

5. **Hotel freebie mini sewing kits** with needles, safety pins, and a variety of basic threads for last-minute button repairs.

6. **Sharpie Permanent Black Marker** makes a great touch up for scuffs on black shoes (even silk or satins), boots, and bags.

7. **Evercare Fabric Shaver** gets rid of pills on sweaters.

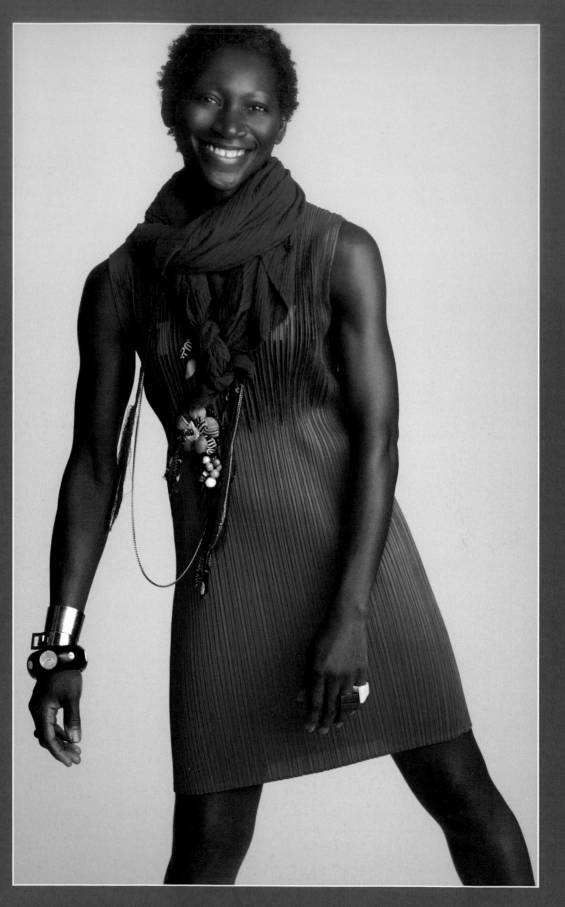

Edris Nicholls
in bright orange
dress, good for
cocktail parties

7. Do a dress rehearsal.

Not kidding! The key to getting fashion looks right is to test them out at home in front of your mirror before you wear them. This saves valuable time and gives you the opportunity to tweak underpinnings and try different combos. When you're rushing to get dressed you really don't have time to swap options or really work on figuring out a look without the pressure of time—especially for events, trips, parties, and social opportunities aside from work. Set aside one long leisurely afternoon every couple of months. This will also give you a chance to evaluate any tailoring needs, shoe repairs, and edit out items that no longer work.

8. Get spray tanned to de-stress big evenings fast.

I'm not a fan of salon spray tans as a lifestyle habit. It's expensive and usually leads to a phony look when done regularly. I much prefer the milder boost of an at-home gradual self-tanner, but the salon spray will provide a little more color everywhere and absolutely evenly.

> A fake tan doesn't hide age and sun damage so much as it blurs skin discolorations thoroughly right down to your toes.

Every once in a while a salon tan can get us confidently past the brown spots, cellulite, loose crepey skin, or vein-y legs our fashion choices expose. It helps those first moments at the beach, on resort vacations, at destination beach weddings, or when you're wearing a sleeveless dress or gown. At home you can maintain the look yourself after the initial pro spray.

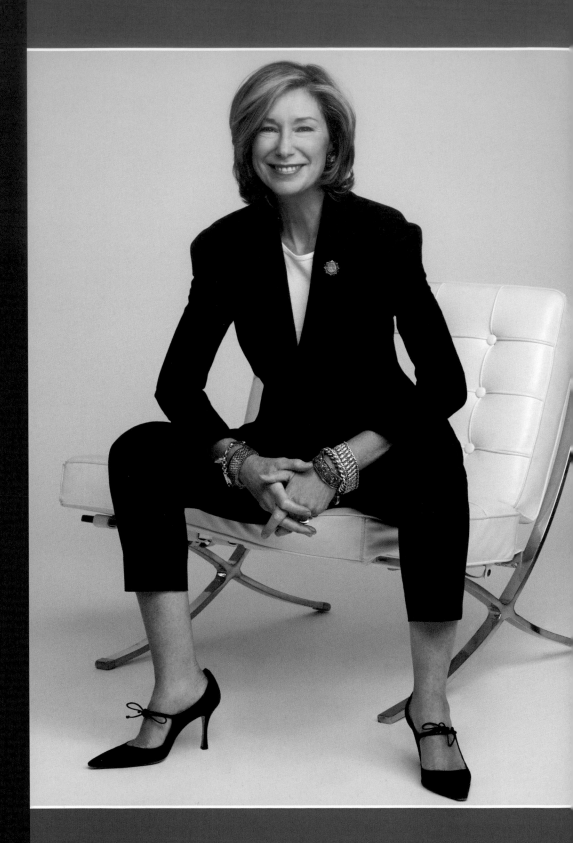

valerie

valerie on:

age and fashion: "I don't buy inexpensive, crappy stuff anymore; only beautiful fabrics and beautifully tailored clothes. I also don't wear anything too revealing. I think a woman my age is sexy when she dresses and behaves in a way that indicates she knows herself. I hate seeing a woman from the back in tight anything, high heels, and long flowing (usually dyed hair) and then she turns around and is thirty years older than you thought she'd be from the back. That mutton-dressed-as-lamb thing to me is very sad."

wardrobe: "When the weather is warm, I wear dresses and skirts with a tee and embellished flat sandals or a simple platform heel if I need to be dressy. In cold weather my favorite pieces are black stretch corduroy skinny jeans, a cashmere sweater, and black suede Jimmy Choo ankle boots with a kitten heel. I have a couple of Chanel pieces I adore, a rust color Hermès blazer I got at a flea market, and a few DVF dresses which fit me like a dream. I'm not label conscious but I am a fan of great fabrics and tailoring."

shopping: "I almost never shop anymore. When I do, here's where I shop: Bergdorf Goodman for dressy stuff, Uniqlo for sporty. The end! I don't shop for clothes online. Twice a year I buy a few things like skirts and tees for summer and then for winter I refresh my cashmeres with a couple more gray or black V-necks or short-sleeve turtlenecks. Every summer I buy a couple pairs of flat sandals and a pair of heels; for winter, one pair of black kitten-heeled ankle boots."

valerie monroe
Beauty Director, *O the Oprah Magazine*

TRADE SECRETS

KNOCK THEIR EYES OUT.

WEAR COSTUME JEWELRY FOR IMPACT. More is more when it comes to jewelry. Every fashion icon from Diana Vreeland to legendary style maven Iris Apfel makes this their motto: Don't blow all the glitz on decorative shoes at night when everyone is talking face to face. Junk jewelry is fun and should be. You need to hit people over the head with one major faux can't-take-my-eyes-off-it necklace, earrings, or giant cocktail rings. Hefty stones and standout stacks of bracelets make any simple dress or top spectacular. Remember at a crowded party or a dinner no one looks down. They focus on you from the waist up.

BE PREPARED FOR THE 24 HOUR DATE.

LAYER AND WEAR FLATS. Chic flats or boots you can walk in and slim cropped pants or jeans are always a good day into night base. Layering allows you to control coverage and build in options for warmth or flattery. If you're newly single, separated, or getting back into dating after 40, know that dating has changed. The old dinner and a movie routine is still alive although the movie might be a four-hour, HD, live-from-the-Met opera. But a date can also mean gallery hopping or a day at the flea market and a bite afterwards if we're still up for it. Date clothes need to be fluid enough to move from one scenario to another without running home to change—unless the "date" is time limited and clearly casual or dressed up.

LET YOUR BODY ROLE-PLAY.

FAKE IT UNTIL YOU MAKE IT REAL. Before a party or a big event we often carry tension and nerves in our shoulders and neck. It affects the fit of your clothes and your body language. Here are my tips: Drop your shoulders. Your chest will automatically look better and your neck longer. For the cocktail part of the evening stand with your weight on one hip and leg and bend the other Instead of planting both feet firmly. Tuck your clutch securely under your left arm and use that hand to hold your drink too. This frees your right hand for shakes, greetings, and makes lean in kisses easier and spill-free. Add a high-gloss or shimmery topcoat and rings that catch the light. You do talk with your hands, don't you?

Nina Griscom, a former top model, knows body language and fashion work together.

NIGHT LIGHT ENCOUR-AGES MORE MAKEUP, COLOR, AND SHIMMER.

TAKE ADVANTAGE OF THE OPPORTUNITY. Evening lighting is soft and diffused. It means you can and should step up everything from makeup to glam clothes and details without fear of overdoing it. Rich jewel tones, candy colors, and bold metallics you might hesitate to wear for day play well in subdued night light. There's one catch: The simpler and more minimalist your clothes, the glitzier, stronger, and more colorful your makeup can be. The more richly textured, layered, colored, or detailed your clothes, the more neutral in color your makeup should be.

WEAR A DRESS WITH SLEEVES IF YOU HATE YOUR ARMS.

Designers have finally caught on to our wish for formal gowns and truly glam dresses that don't force us to bare our arms. The booming category of evening dresses—long and short—with sleeves and in lots of cases higher necklines, is a great idea. Centuries away from the dowdy, frumpy puff-sleeve ball gowns of the past, these sleek styles have a purely contemporary look.

LOOK FOR FITTED SLEEVES, A BODY-SKIMMING SHAPE AND HIGH NECKLINE CUT STRAIGHT ACROSS LIKE A BOATNECK, SLIGHTLY OFF SHOULDER, OR CUT IN A WIDE V.

They range from low-cost stunners by Lauren Ralph Lauren, and Calvin Klein in the $190 range to $1,600 for a black sequin-covered, long sleeve gown by Diane von Furstenberg that's a drop-dead evening version of her signature style. All you have to add with a gown like that are strappy sandals and sparkling earrings.

WORK THE LOCATION. MIAMI, KANSAS CITY, AND CHICAGO HAVE DIFFERENT VIBES.

When I travel for parties and weddings I always feel too dressed up in LA, too drab in Miami, and too clearly like a New York girl in Dallas or Santa Fe. The light changes, the atmosphere alters and the personality of where you are differs. They all have a lot to do with what you wear. The choice between a neutral or color, solid or print, tailored or soft, is influenced by location. In New York, anything I wear—from matte jersey to sequins—looks and feels best in neutrals. Festivities out of town mean hitting my closet for color or metallics.

JERSEY IS A MAJOR PLAYER WHEN IT COMES TO VERSATILITY ANYWHERE IN THE WORLD.

You can't beat it for a destination wedding, a vacation where a great evening-out dress is part of the plan or simply when you're the hostess of a party or an actual event yourself. Draped, shirred, or wrapped jersey in any color or print is comfortable, easy to move in, hides tummy bloat, and won't crease. You can always relax and add some serious shapewear beneath to keep an eye on jiggles and flab. At the high end, no one does it better than Donna Karan but try Tadashi Shoji, Maggy London, and Adrianna Papell for more affordable options.

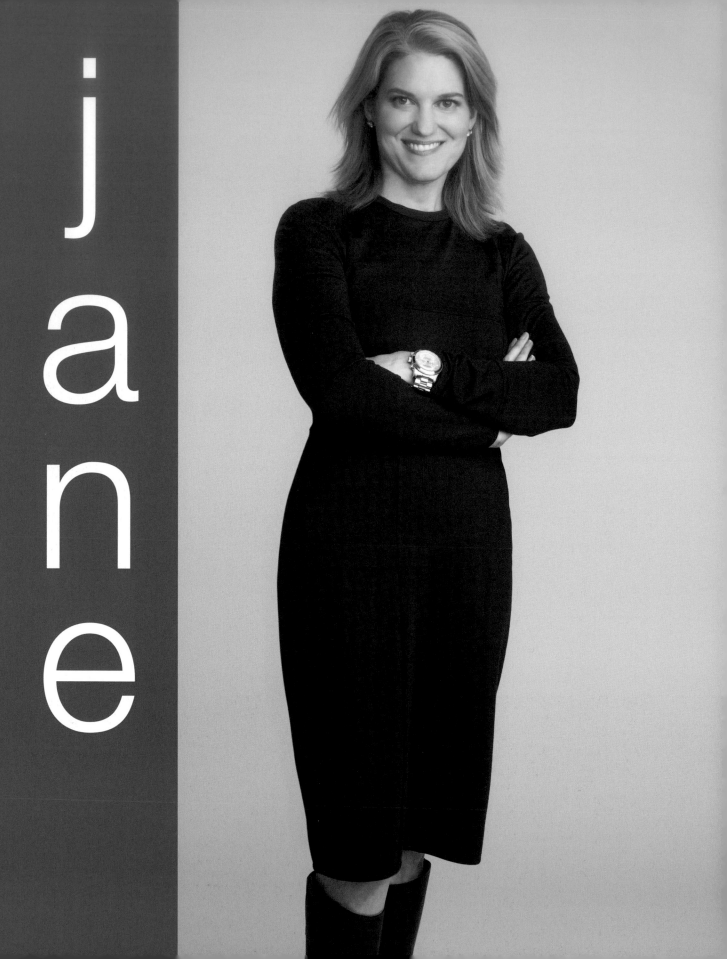

j
a
n
e

jane on:

shopping: "I'm skilled at buying without even trying stuff on and I've had great luck at sample sales and on eBay. I get the biggest shopping thrill when I find a great Jil Sander dress on eBay for under $300, and it's happened a lot. My tip: Know the designer, know your size. I rarely buy full price and almost always wait for the big sales at Bergdorf's or Barneys. Plus I always shop at Uniqlo, H&M, and Zara."

age and fashion: "In the past couple of years I've decided my legs are no longer suitable for show above the knee, so my dresses are longer. My arms have become flabby so the sleeveless dresses and tops that I loved forever are worn significantly less. There is definitely such a thing as age-appropriate fashion. Since I'm at least ten years older than most of my friends, every once in a while I look at some dress and boots outfit I'm wearing and say to myself, "Should a woman close to 50 be wearing a schoolgirl dress?" Not a slutty dress, mind you, but rather a prim and child-like one. I often wonder if I dress too young, but rarely do I give a damn."

jane larkworthy
Executive Beauty Director, *W* magazine

I'm Obsessed with . . .

Here are fifteen of the most confusing, irritating situations women 40+ face. Some of them, like galas, fundraisers, and mother-of-the bride weddings, have evolved with age; others grow out of new social situations like divorce, remarriage, or relocation to a new climate. Any situation is a potential social or business meeting, from a morning with your pup at the dog run, cocktails with the girls, or taking part in a charity walk-a-thon.

Dress for it!

Black-tie friends and family wedding: You can go long or knee-length here. If you go short, make it an ultra-dressy fabric like silk taffeta, lace, or satin with details like beading or draping. Don't try to get by in a basic tailored LBD with dressy shoes and bag. **A one-shoulder knee-length dress or a sequined long sleeve shift can take the stuffiness out of the night.** Fancy slim heels that sparkle and a small, structured evening bag are essential.

Dating after divorce: Some women divorce husbands after twenty-five years of marriage, others are on their second or third time around. Some now prefer men young enough to be their sons; others seek men the same age who share a similar history and references. Getting back into the single life after a long-term marriage or the most recent one is a chance to reinvent your look and step up the glamour. **Get new jeans, fresh heels, a body-skimming dress and sweaters with V-necks to replace your walk-the-dog bootcuts, clogs, and fleece.** Start getting manicures and pedicures again and consider beachy highlights to brighten up your hair and face.

What to Wear for the Time of My Life!

Dating a younger guy: You're a woman with a past! Whether your new type is an academic, baker, fireman, photographer, or cosmetic surgery resident you need clothes that look more contemporary without changing your style. **Think Demi Moore, Madonna, Susan Sarandon, Goldie Hawn, and Julianne Moore here for inspiration.** Show your shape, legs, or arms with body-skimming clothes, sleeveless dresses, and skirts, as often as possible.

Dressing for the gym or health club: Women new to the workout scene may not realize the social implications and benefits extend way beyond flattening your tummy and toning your legs. These venues are ways to meet new friends and potential dating material. If you've relocated to a new neighborhood this is social-life central. Your shredded old leggings and stained Rolling Stones tee are not okay. Pull your hair back in a ponytail or wear a black stretch headband at the hairline to keep locks off your sweaty face. No scrunchies—use plain elastic in black or matched to your hair color. **Wear clingy matte black workout clothes— they make everyone look more buff and serious about fitness.** Skip the visors that easily add twenty years to your look.

Funeral/wake: You want to dress modestly and not call attention to your clothes or yourself for once. Choose a black jacket and pants or pencil skirt, a high-neck black dress with some sort of sleeve or a coat (could be a black trench). **Add low heels that allow you to walk to the grave site, dark glasses so you can grieve without worrying about your eye makeup running.** Minimal jewelry is okay; pearls always work.

Getting married for the first time: If you've never been married before you might be tempted by a big-deal gown, complete with fairytale veil and train. Let's cut to the chase. Skip anything too girly or too retro after 40. No Victorian-esque virginal gowns, no full skirt with crinolines or strapless corsets with layers of tulle. **If you're doing a long gown at all, make it simple and sleek—a column, a subtle A-line, a one-shoulder silhouette. Otherwise, wear a tailored sheath.** Celebs who have married for the first time after forty (like Ellen DeGeneres, Salma Hayek, and Elizabeth Hurley) have influenced the bridal market to riff on fashionable elegant evening clothes. Even a white tux could be an elegant choice for a certain woman with style.

Getting married again: This could be your second, third, or fourth time around. I married at twenty-four, thirty-four, and fifty-four, and every time the dress and the wedding got more casual and more intimate. The first time I wore a white Jax wedding gown with a bohemian look I'd seen in *Vogue* and had a huge garden wedding at my parents' home. Wedding #2 I wore an ankle-length ivory cashmere knit sweater-dress (made for the occasion) with a long cashmere scarf and the wedding party was a few friends and my daughter Jen. The third time around was at the local justice of the peace and it was just my husband, myself, and two witnesses we grabbed in the court. **I wore a silver-sequin covered pencil skirt and a white cashmere V-neck sweater with silver sandals and you know what . . . I was just as happy in that.** What's my point? It all depends on you—anything goes and you don't have to wear white. The time of day or night is not an issue. A big old wedding in a ballroom with four hundred guests at night is going to require a lot more dressing than a quiet ceremony and lunch for twenty.

Going back to college: Whether you're auditing classes or going for a degree, being surrounded by students will make you want to fit in. Don't fall into the trap of trying to be one of them—they know you're not. **Wear jeans, khakis, cargos, flats, layered to go in neutrals and don't forget the cool modern glasses.** A messenger bag or hobo, not a backpack, looks right.

High school/college reunion:
Every single woman wants to look thinner and more youthful for her reunions. As tempting as it may be to do the LBD dress for its pound-paring abilities, be careful which one you choose. Don't do the Robert Palmer "Addicted to Love" look of tight black dress, red lips, and stilettos. Don't wear any dress with a neckline that could result in a wardrobe malfunction. Tacky! Expectations run high at these events and you do want your old boyfriend's jaw to drop even if you're happily married—well, especially then! Reunions are sometimes a one-shot festive evening or a weekend marathon of casual and formal. For the party, a cocktail look is what you're after. **A shapely dress in a gorgeous fun color like shocking pink, fuchsia, or orange makes you easy to spot** but a festive print or an LBD could certainly work too. For a weekend-long celebration, I'd also bring a pencil and body-filled cashmere with a belt, slim cropped pants, and jeans with V-neck cardigans.

Mother-of-the-bride:
No one ever wants to be cliché, so don't fall into the lavender chiffon and ruffles trap. You're in the #2 spot here! Depending on the formality or informality of the wedding, go long or short. Discuss privately with the bride her thoughts and preferences in terms of color and style but stick to your guns when it comes to selecting the actual dress. **I'd root for a sleek one-shoulder or body-skimming column here.** This gives you a lot of room to maneuver around the color theme and fit with a little draping. Nothing fussy, frilly, retro, or full.

Moving to Florida:
If you're moving to any hot climate from a cold, multi-season urban setting, brighten or lighten up. Don't feel you have to lose the one-color or neutral core strategy.

Add more white to any of your blacks, navys, and grays to brighten them, or select more colorful prints that contain your base colors when buying new pieces. Add larger solid items in color to complement the accessories and basics you own. Warm corals, reds, and pinks, look great with all your whites, browns, and beiges. Cool cobalt-blues, violets, and fuchsias team up well with blacks, navys, and grays.

Pregnant after 40: Show off your bump with stretchy, comfy jersey tops and dresses. Draped necklines, ruching, and raised waists mold to evolving curves and look more contemporary than loose tailored shifts and shirts on mature women. Prints add style and variety—just aim for artsy modern rather than dainty florals. Wear thin layers for comfort control. Leggings and pretty flats (feet will swell) balance fullness above with a lean line hips down.

Tourist: This is where the 40+ crowd of American women always get a bad rap and it's about time it stops. We're experienced, sophisticated travelers so just to review the top points: Neutral colors in layers strip off or pile on easily and look fashionable in Paris or Big Sur. Cropped jeans or slim cropped pants mean no problem stepping in puddles or dragging pants through dirt and street grime. Wearing comfortable flats, Converse or similar style sneakers make walking easy. Choose sneakers/hiking boots for serious sporty trips. Lightweight cross-body messenger bags keep our hands free, our stuff secure, and make stashing maps, guidebooks, tickets, and passports easy. A big scarf, a cardigan, and a print skirt go a long way towards dressing up tees and layers. Oversized sunglasses boost wrinkle protection and make eye contact with strangers comfortable. You can repeat the same outfit seven times. Unless you're under surveillance no one is keeping score or notices even on a group tour.

Sports event: Going to your grandson's baseball games or seeing the Yankees in action means layers, comfort, and sun protection. **Jeans and slim cropped pants, layers you can peel off or add on at will, a baseball cap or knit beanie (depending on the season), flats, and sunglasses are the recipe.** I went to my first Yankees game at fifty-eight and wished I had brought a heavier sweater (as the day cooled down) and wore looser, softer jeans instead of tight skinnies and boots—FYI.

Your Internet photo: How to look great for a picture everyone will see on Facebook, match.com, or in your LinkedIn headshot? Don't use an old photo—some detail will give it a way or people will suspect it's old. **Wear a neck-lengthening, fitted top in a solid color and contemporary shape.** You don't want to add bulk to the neck, shoulders, or upper arms. A tailored dress, classy white shirt (unbuttoned to a V, sleeves pushed up for attitude), a fitted tee, or a knit V-neck sweater will always look more youthful and friendly than a jacket. If you do wear a jacket (let's say for a corporate head shot) be sure it's updated, fitted, and has slim sleeves and a high armhole. Wear it over something casual like a tank to elongate the neck.

When it comes to the pose, angle one shoulder towards the camera and turn your head slightly off-center so your "good" side is also towards the camera. You don't want to be head-on straight, mug-shot style. Be candid and as relaxed as possible. Pay attention to where the light hits your face and tilt your chin up slightly and project it out and forward to avoid shadows. If the lens is below your eye level you'll have a photo with a double chin (count on it). Make sure the lens of the camera is level with your eyes or above you. Close your eyes for a few seconds and yawn to relax your face before the shot. Don't hesitate to ask the photographer to wait while you do this warm up. Models do it between shots all the time.

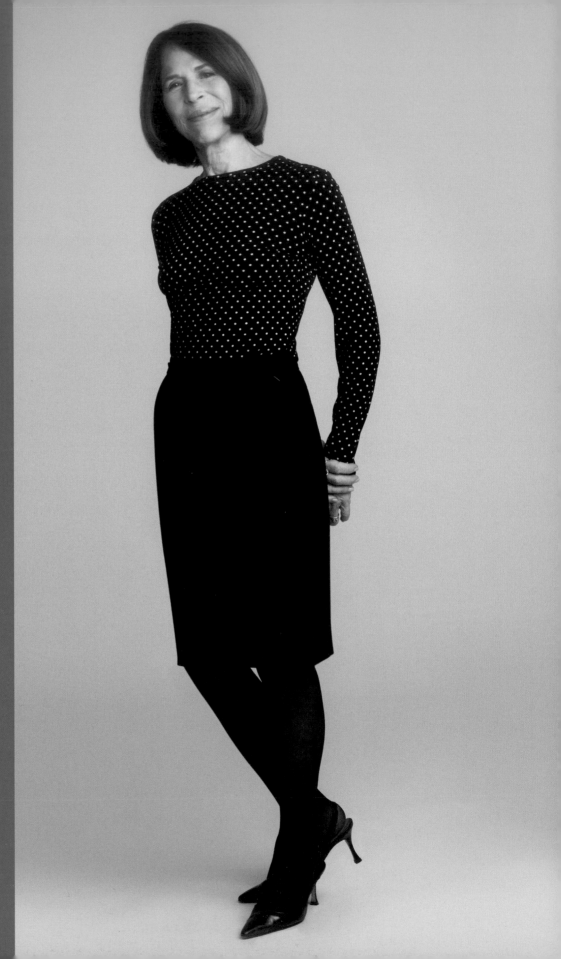

marilyn

marilyn on:

style:
"My personal style has always been understated. I'm a firm believer in less is more! What's important to me is good fit, beautiful, natural fabrics and a graceful line. I'm most comfortable in neutral colors. Occasionally, I'll wear a great red or orange jacket or red shoes for fun and surprise!"

age and fashion:
"I like to look my best whether I'm wearing an agnès b. dress or French jeans, but I wouldn't wear what a thirty-year-old wears. I prefer modesty while still subtly revealing my shape and legs. That means well-fitting, fairly covered-up tops, shapely skirts that fall to the middle of my knees or slightly lower (never shorter), and pants that are slightly flared but never baggy. I walk, do weight bearing exercise and yoga, eat small, healthy meals five times a day, drink lots of water and this routine has enabled me to stay slim and fit so I can wear the kinds of clothes I prefer. Being responsible for your body pays off in health and fashion benefits."

real life:
"I spend a great deal of time in my art studio so I'm usually in khakis and long sleeve tees which I layer for warmth and style, and clogs which are comfortable and make me feel taller. It's all very informal but when the occasion arises I love to get dressed up, too!"

marilyn glass
Artist

CHAPTER SEVEN

FASHIONABLY FURIOUS

Road rage? How about fashion rage? We wonder sometimes if stores and designers really understand our purchase power.

The biggest complaint about fashion I hear from women 40+ is that designers seem more interested in dressing younger women and celebrities than us! Of course economic strategies and media opportunities are partly to blame for the shift in focus, but we're too big and powerful a group to ignore. We're firecrackers who live busy, multi-dimensional lives that require style and updates of basics. Despite our grievances and frustrations we still love fashion and shopping. We have money from years of work and smart investments (and in some cases inheritances or divorce settlements) and need more wearable choices at every price level to help us stay in the game. The bonus of staying healthy and fit now is being able to wear whatever we want whenever we want. Fashion will always have the ability to make us feel great even as our bodies and lifestyles change. We sit in movie theaters and check sales on our iPads instead of watching the trailers; we shop for dresses online at 1 a.m. and try on every shoe in the department waiting for the sales associate to find the "other" shoe. We're picky and practical but boy do we love clothes.

Dianne Vavra

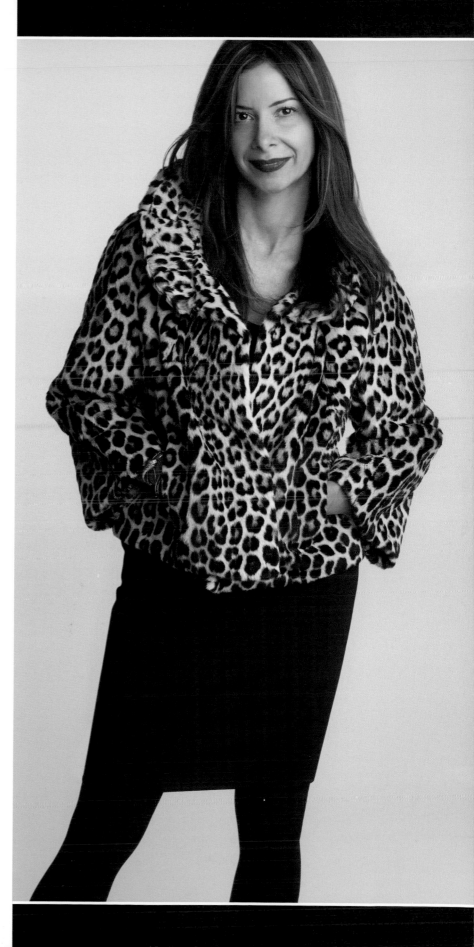

Here's the real backstory

In the last ten years fashion has become a super-sized global business. Designers now get their inspiration from street style, new technology, fabric innovations, historical archives of designers' past, world news, sports, music, and of course the new generation of fashionable young women who love to show their bodies and skin. Like designers, we've evolved too and have become a generation of know-it-alls who are influenced by everything we see, read, and hear. Here are the new facts of life:

- **Most women 40+ do not live in the fashion spotlight or work in a business where wearing the hottest trends validates them.** We just want clothes with a dose of fashion. When most fashion magazines do editorial features that show "real women" and the clothes they actually wear, those photographed are usually in a related fashion/publishing/entertainment business, work for the magazine, or are some sort of a celebrity. Unless of course they're talking about weight issues, and then "authentic" women are used for the before and afters. But you knew that.

- **Most women 40+ are black belt shoppers who know what they want and just need help finding it.** They don't need advice on what's new in the entire store or sixteen items to go with the item they are seeking. They just need a go and get it, eager-to-help salesperson.

- **Most women 40+ say they feel ignored by sales help who pander to younger consumers.** They give up and leave the store because the routine makes them angry. They're reluctant to shop where they feel marginalized.

- **Most women 40+ like to shop alone.** The pack mentality leaves at about age thirty and we don't need our husbands, boyfriends, friends, or daughters to give a thumbs-up. This makes shopping so pleasurable—we're in a bubble for a few minutes or an hour . . . alone.

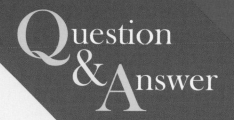

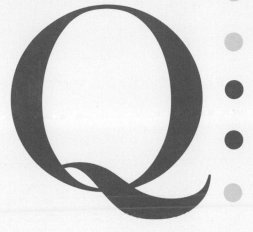

Q: What's a happy fashion moment these days?

A: When I emerge from the dressing room or my closet feeling comfortable, classy, and chic, instead of frustrated, frumpy, and fed up.

Clothes say it for us. Instead of tattoos and piercings we do fashion. Well some of us do all three, but for the most part we want our style to say who we are. In this chapter we'll solve the style taboos and dilemmas we're dying to talk about.

What fashion mood management can do for you now

As consumers we live in a fast-paced world where the motto is "more is more." We're encouraged to shop every single day online and in stores with e-mail alerts, markdowns, and sales that occur more frequently. Fashion is fabulous but it also has become a pretty stressful experience for lots of women. The emotional intensity of shopping and dressing varies from relaxing to distressing, ecstatic to maddening. We're disappointed when we try on something new and it's more unflattering than we anticipated from the photo.

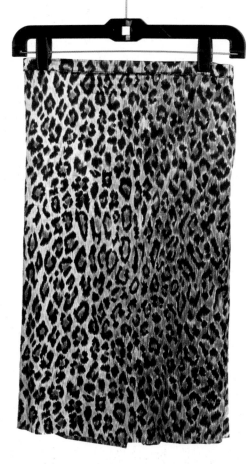

We're happy when we grab "the last one." We're thrilled when a salesperson locates that dress we want at another store and says "I'll have it sent in your size with no extra charge from Hawaii." Positive shopping and dressing is a mood booster, negative shopping and dressing is not. It can cause our heart rate and blood pressure to accelerate, along with the stress hormone cortisol. Fortunately there are smart, easy solutions to stabilizing style and shopping for all of us.

Me too! Same thing!

I was spoiled by my years as a fashion editor. All that hanging out with designers, stylists, and PR and fashion execs made it too easy. My idea of shopping was snagging finds at designer sample sales and ordering privately straight from designer line sheets or showroom racks. When I re-entered the real world of clothes and shopping the reality shock was acute. Part of it was of course that I knew too much but part of it was age. Without my meticulous pre-edits as a magazine editor, shopping became a real drag.

Browsing on the Internet became my favorite strategy and still is. It enables me to preview and edit quickly and effortlessly order items from brands I love without a lot of drama. But I still crave the in-store experience. There's something about being able to touch, see, handle, and try on the clothes that I need. Occasionally there are blips. Recently a twenty-ish sales assistant advised me (unasked): "Don't worry. You're not too old for that dress; you have a great body and anyway you're going to wear a cardigan over it, right?" You've probably been there too, haven't you?

Cynde Watson

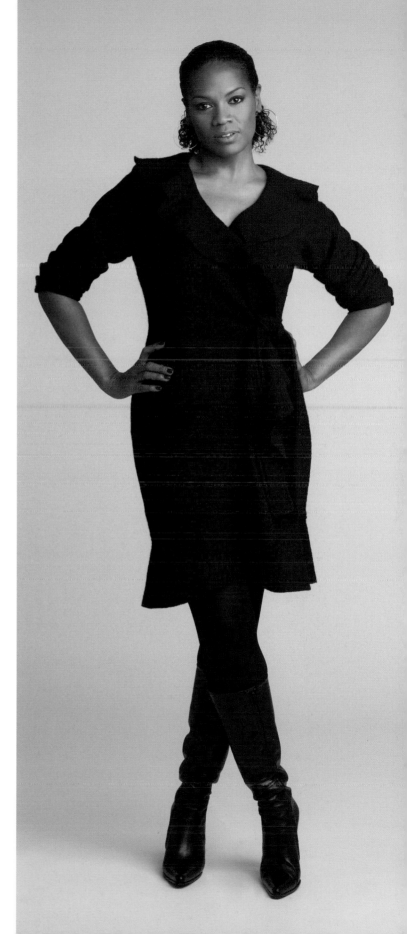

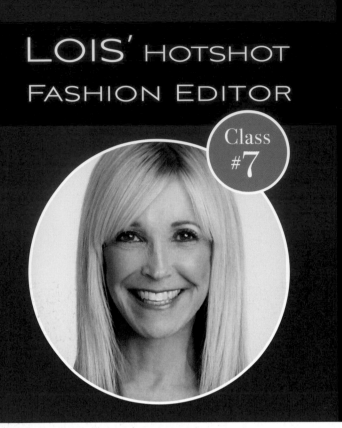

LOIS' HOTSHOT FASHION EDITOR

Class #7

10 Secrets To Getting The Clothes You Need And Want

1. Shop online more.

We're all urbanized now, no matter where we live.

Women living in small, rural or suburban towns now shop and dress like their peers in the big cities. Online shopping has made boundaries between rural, urban, and suburban obsolete. The hottest runway trends and brands are accessible to us all on the Internet. Even if you don't live in a big city or near a major mall you can shop for Diane von Furstenberg dresses, J.Crew sweaters, Zara jackets, and Stuart Weitzman shoes. What's not to love? There's no hunting for a parking spot, no dealing with indifferent or inattentive

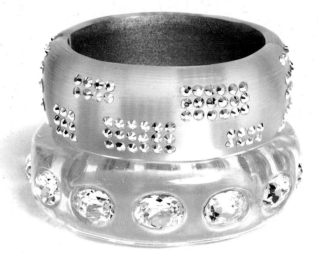

salespeople, no waiting for a dressing room or standing in a long line to pay, no need to send someone looking for another size in the stockroom, no need to get dressed, put on makeup, go out in the rain, snow or humidity, and wreck your blowout.

If you've been conditioned to think online shopping is hit or miss, I disagree! There has been enormous improvement in the amount of information and online presentation, from exact specifications about fit, to videos of the item on a moving model and views of the item from every possible angle. Most department store sites say exactly how long a dress or skirt is from the natural waist or tell you the length of a jacket or top from shoulder to hem. This helps you gauge fit when you know the model is 5'11" and wearing a size 4, the item is shown on a mannequin, or the photo itself is cropped.

You can fill up and modify your shopping bag or cart over several days, unlike stores that are now reluctant to "hold" merchandise.

You can comparison shop several stores for similar items at the same time and track items as they go on sale. My favorite part is checking reviews from women who bought the items and online exclusives that wouldn't be available in the store itself anyway. Net-a-porter.com, the most luxurious of the fashion retail sites delivers your purchase to your door gift wrapped as if you were a celebrity, and the customer service makes you feel like you're calling from the Ritz in Paris instead of your bedroom.

2. Shop alone. Your best personal shopper is you.

No one else can ever know or understand your frustrations and the way you feel about clothes and your body as it ages and changes. Shopping may be retail therapy for you but it's not group therapy. It's like any relationship. Only you can appreciate how a weight gain or loss influences your options. Only you really understand your obsession with the fit of Theory pants or your addiction to anything striped.

Make a list of what you wear the most, want the most, and need the most. Do they match up? The closer you can get the better.

Fashion with its blustering bi-polar exclamations (in/out! love it/hate it! get it/toss it!) and self-important decrees ("Yellow is the new black.") is there only for your personal entertainment and a few useful suggestions. Never ask a sales assistant how she thinks you look in something. It's her job to encourage you to spend, regardless if she makes a commission or is paid hourly. Trust your gut.

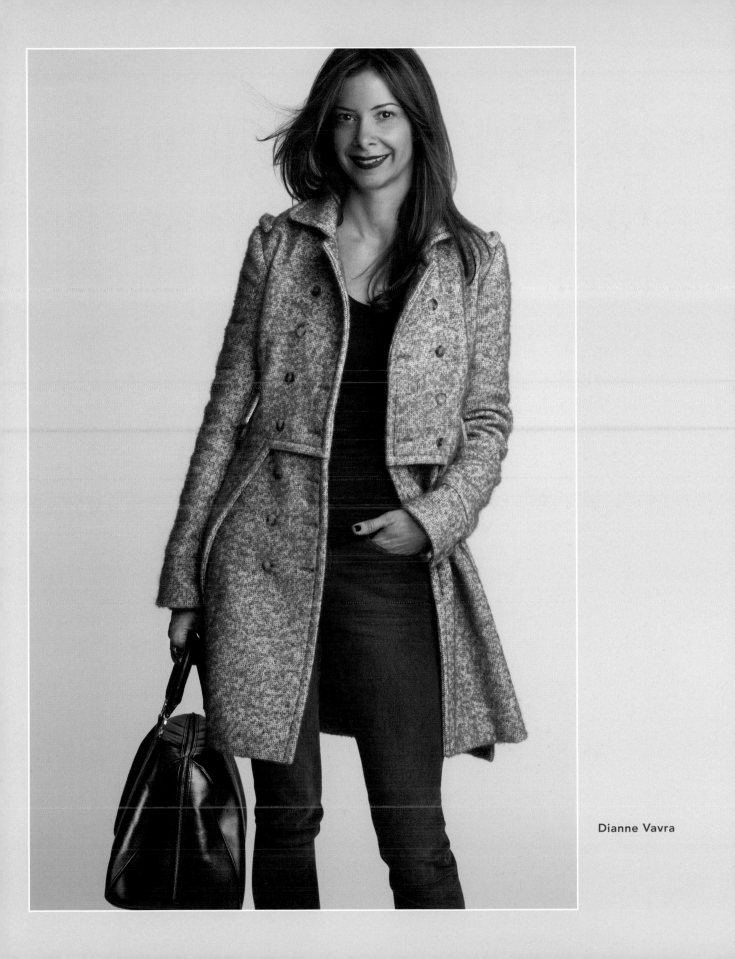

Dianne Vavra

3. Service matters.
Expect it or demand it. Taking charge

of your shopping perks is one way to de-stress the process. My sister Rebecca calls customer service and asks for free shipping if it's not offered online. Know what? She gets it! She does this even when she's spending under the amount specified to qualify for free shipping. Sure she's a hotshot lawyer and a shrewd negotiator but she's also a smart consumer, and in a tough competitive economy that's being strategic.

Alterations are a big deal for us too and they do become more essential as we age. When I shop department stores or specialty stores, first thing I ask is, "Does the store have a tailor/seamstress on staff and available right now and is tailoring free?" Frankly I'd rather have this service than a café overlooking the cashmeres or all the gift-with purchases offered at the cosmetic counters.

**Get a sense of entitlement about alterations,
free shipping, discounts, and customer service in general.**

4. Let someone
else do the research.

Don't drive yourself crazy. Let customer service find those items you desperately want. They can locate clothing items and accessories that are sold out locally or on the website. They will even waive shipping fees to get them to you.

Take advantage of any online personal shopper offers to help (with a pop-up box or a link). They can provide extra details about items you're considering that are not included in the description.

Sometimes photos can be deceptive or tricky. Customer service or an online personal shopper, also known as "Live Chat," can reveal what's not shown. This is especially important for sale items and online exclusives you can't try on in stores. Customer service can tell you how "stilled" items (anything photographed flat instead of on a model) really fit. You can find out the true color of a shade called bright emerald on screen but appears to be aqua. J.Crew customer service helped me understand the exact fit and size of a slouchy raglan sleeve top that was an online exclusive and I ended up ordering two.

5. Buy midway trends.

After 40 you don't want the trendiest of the trends in your closet or on your body. As each designer gets on board the trend-of-the-season bandwagon the exact degree of trendiness will vary. Let's say stripes, peplums, and metallics are hot—you could wear a striped dress or a peplum blouse or a metallic bag, but a metallic striped peplum dress? No way do you need that!

Any trendy item works in one of three ways: It can be fairly classic with a touch of trend, more contemporary with a slightly trendier look or flat out super-trendy. Know your limit.

6. Stick to brands and stores that are "you."

This prevents letdowns and shop-pping setbacks. Knowing which brands suit your style, shape, and price range makes online shopping pretty foolproof.

Just eliminate the labels and stores that no longer work for your wallet, body, and lifestyle (even if they have for years) and identify the new ones that do. Post the list on a sticky above your computer.

Letting go of old favorite brands or stores is like a breakup or divorce—you can't force fashion when it no longer works and there are plenty of new choices. Don't fight it. Instead, start "dating" new sites and labels to find the ones that deliver the fit, proportions, information, attitude, affordability, and attention you need. Some brand names kept coming up as I interviewed women. Those that appeal to us now across the board for a variety of reasons are Zara, Tory Burch, Diane von Furstenberg, J.Crew, Theory, MICHAEL Michael Kors, Rachel Roy, Milly, Lauren by Ralph Lauren and Ann Taylor. The skirt lengths, prices, color choices, and fit of the pants and dresses have a lot to do with why these are favorites.

7. Comfort's great but don't stop there.

Comfort is a word that comes up a lot when we talk about fashion but it doesn't mean living in sweats and sneakers 24/7. Women want to keepthe fashion lose the aches and hassle of clothes that constrict movement or (let's be honest) breathing and standing. Never give up fashion for comfort because you don't need to.

Here are the top comfort fashions to own:

Chic pumps with extra padding and a comfortable pitch: Like those by Stuart Weitzman and Cole Haan

Soft moccasins, driving shoes, and boat shoes: Like those by Sperry Top-Sider, Jack Rogers, Ugg Australia, and Hunter

Ballet flats: Like those by Tory Burch, KORS Michael Kors, and Stuart Weitzman

Classy sneakers: Like those by Converse, Superga, and Vans

Long soft silky tanks and tees: In cotton and rayon jersey or modal, like those by Gap and J.Crew

Slim comfy ankle cropped pants: Like those by J.Jill, Ann Taylor, J.Crew, Banana Republic, Theory

Tunic blouses: Like those by Tory Burch, J.Jill

Ponte knit pants, skirts, dresses, and jackets: Like clothes by J.Jill, Lands' End, Talbots, Not Your Daughter's Jeans

Relaxed (but not big or sloppy) flat-knit sweaters: Including those that cover our rears or have a subtle A-shape fit, like those by Eileen Fisher, J.Jill, Uniqlo, and J.Crew

Jersey dresses: Like those by Diane von Furstenberg, Target

Waterproof leather and suede flat boots: Like those by Stuart Weitzman, Aquatalia

Long and draped cardigans: Like those by Eileen Fisher, Inhabit, J.Jill

Soft relaxed jeans: Like those by Levi's, Gap, Current/Elliott

Wire-free, hard-working support bras: Like those by Playtex, Bali, Wacoal

8. Never worry if you look younger or thinner than anyone else . . . or your former self.

We've spent decades comparing ourselves to friends, relatives, neighbors, colleagues, celebrities, models, and random people on the street. This was (we now admit) unrealistic but we couldn't help ourselves. Most women grow out of this competitive state by the time they reach 40—definitely by 45. Now we have a new threat to our self-confidence. The fashion industry has started using computer-generated images to advertise clothes. Frankly, I'm all for seeing a little imperfection myself.

By now you have better things to think about and any style doubts you may have can be solved with the lessons in this book.

9. Stop passive-aggressive fashion behavior. So chums lose the hostility and confront store managers and customer service execs nicely but firmly about your concerns and disappointment in them. Take a time-out—sip a latte. Then give useful, clear helpful suggestions like, "I'd love to see more knee-length skirts because the fit of your pencils is incredible except they're

six inches too short and sitting in them is impossible." Follow up with e-mails to key executives. Don't know who they are? Just Google the brand. Believe me, those in charge do want to know why they are losing customers. Forget about getting angry and get constructive.

10. Shop mindfully.

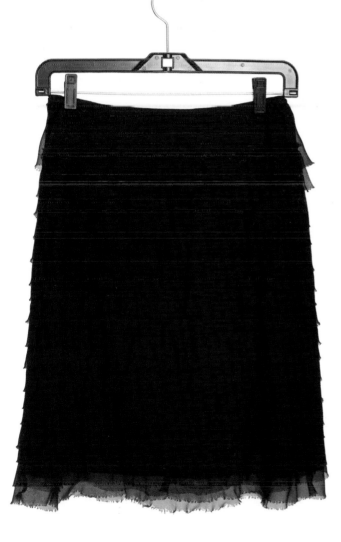

For lots of us, shopping is like being on cruise control. The aisles and racks or clicks whiz by in a blur of color and pattern till something catches our eye. Stylists treat shopping like they're profilers for the FBI and you can too.

Look for wardrobe freshening items that are often shoved in between the same old predictable ones.

Think twice. Would nude pumps with a wedge or platform update your look and lengthen your legs just as well as your usual classic nude pumps? Would a pair of slim tuxedo pants in red instead of the usual black give you a quick dress-up option? Would a sequin-covered bolero instead of a black cardigan make a bare LBD wearable again and give it a shot of glam?

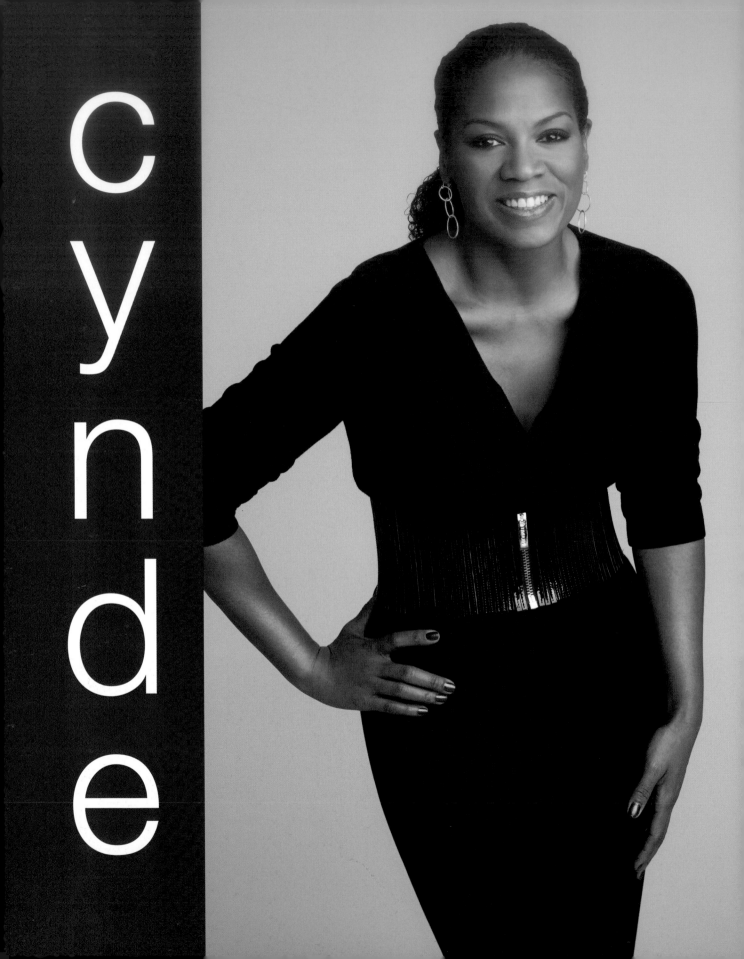

cynde

cynde on:

inspiration:
"I get ideas looking at trends in fashion magazines, celebrity photos, and watching awards shows. It's partly business research and influences my day-to-day work as a makeup and beauty pro. However it doesn't change my overall personal style or my confidence about what works best for me."

wardrobe:
"More dresses! I don't like to spend a lot of time putting looks together and if one piece can make a sleek, fashionable statement and look special, that's all I need. I'm tall and have firm model-y curves, so knits and jersey wrap dresses really do work for my body and are comfortable for work or travel. When I'm on the road for business I need to be able to step off the plane and head straight into a meeting or the studio looking flawless and professional. I like to play up my waist with statement belts—the bolder the better—as part of my signature look. My closet is mostly black with shots of red so everything works together. When I do wear pants or skirts, an elegant crisp white shirt is all I need."

cynde watson

Creator of Color by Cynde Watson,
makeup artist, and beauty entrepreneur

Trade Secrets

Shop in the A.M.

The staff is alert, perky from breakfast and their first shot of caffeine, and the clothes are better organized and neatly displayed. This is the time of day when sales help are most receptive to questions and requests for help.

Shop on vacation or business trips.

You'll find merchandise you can't find at home. You can even avoid paying a higher sales tax in some states. Since major store buyers select specific items from a designer's seasonal lineup to accommodate the tastes of their core customer and pass on others, you may find styles from the collection not available in your own local stores. For example, in the South you will always find more color and a wider selection of feminine styles.

Ask for a discount if you pay in cash.

Smaller stores and boutiques often will give you this courtesy, especially if you are a frequent customer. Speak up! For you paying in cash means no credit card fees and for the vendor less paperwork.

CREATE AN IN-STORE FRIEND.

WHEN APPROACHED BY A SALESPERSON, SMILE AND SAY "HI! I'D LOVE TO LOOK AROUND FIRST BUT I'LL GET BACK TO YOU."

Don't say, "I'm just looking" (even if you are). Asking for a salesperson's card is a great way to build a store insider relationship. When I was looking for a certain item at Barneys, a lovely sales assistant followed me around from item to item. Although I prefer shopping alone, I asked her what she thought of the new store redesign, the brand I was buying, and what she was wearing. She not only tracked down the item I wanted in my size but said it should be marked down on sale.

Marilyn Glass

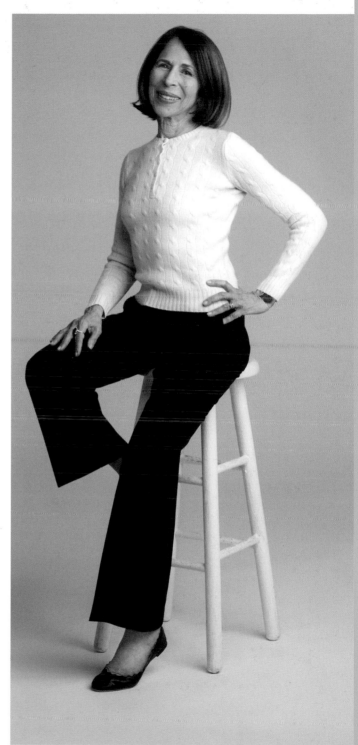

I'm Obsessed with . . .

Salespeople are more interested in helping younger customers. Know this complaint is common among your peers and has nothing to do with you personally. Sure it's annoying when you're ready to buy a $500 dress and the salesperson is chatting to another sales associate about last night, texting, or holding a cell to her ear. Be upfront right from the start.

Smile and say, "Listen, I really need someone to give me personal attention, stick with me while I shop—and be available to find other sizes or items if I need them. Are you the right person for me?"

Why are skirts and dresses from lots of contemporary designers so short?

It seems like luxury brands and super-classic labels are the only ones making knee-ish lengths. Can't contemporary designers offer minis and to the top of the knee? I hear this gripe a lot. There are a lot of great dresses we'd buy if only they were two inches longer.

Why do designers do faux wraps when they can do real ones? Both work for different bodies but offer the same body-defining boost. Faux wrap jersey dresses are speedy to slip on and eliminate the need to wrap and tie so some women just like the ease. The faux crossover design (also called a surplice wrap) can add subtle shape to a blurry middle yet provide the same neck and body lengthening benefit as a true wrap.

Fake wraps are great if you don't actually have a waist.

If you do have a good waistline, a faux wrap won't flatter you. Since it can't be adjusted, the fit will feel too loose through the middle even if it fits at the bust and hip.

My Shopping Issues!

Jeans tags that say "dye transfers if washed with other items" and "don't put these jeans in the dryer" are annoying. The wash before wearing warning on super-saturated, over-dyed dark jeans means exactly that. You don't want the tan leather seats in your car, your good beige bag, or your white sofa stuck with indigo stains, do you? Wash dark jeans in cold water separately—even apart from other jeans and dark tees a dozen times before risking a dark mixed laundry. Test for color fastness by rubbing the jeans over an old white tee.

The shrinkage problem with stretch jeans and the dryer exasperates us too. We don't have the time (or patience) to air-dry and know full-time drying will make jeans too tight to wear. Here's the solution: throw them in the dryer for no more than five to seven minutes and then air-dry the rest.

Chic leather bags that say "Do not get wet. Dye may transfer." can't possibly be true. I bought a famous designer hobo in red leather on sale two years ago and figured the tag was exaggerating the non-color-fast claim. It wasn't. One damp rainy day everything it touched turned blotchy pink. Take any new bags that have dye transfer potential to a shoe repair shop before removing the tags to see if waterproofing is possible. If there is no way to make the bag more resistant to moisture, return before removing the tags. Who needs bag stress?

Undies and tights that specify hand wash. Yes this is maddening. When it comes to inexpensive thongs and boy shorts or bikinis, ignore the wash-by-hand cautions. You do need to make the extra effort with bras and tights and pricier undies so they will not lose their hold or shape, snag, pill, or bag. Soak them in the sink with a swish of baby shampoo, bath gel, or a special rinse made for hand washing delicates. Add a dab of your favorite scent to the water or the damp garments themselves as they dry.

Size varies brand to brand, designer to designer, store to store. Yup, there is absolutely no standardization of size. But be realistic—how can there be regulation when our bodies are so diverse? You can be a size 8 and 5'3" or 5'7". You can be an 8 and have a 34 B chest or a 34 D, a trim waist or none, be short or long waisted. Get over it and learn which brands or designers work for your body.

Petites are not miniature women. We all know by now petite refers to a stature that is 5'4" or less, any size. The variations of bodies that are considered petite are endless. Some shorter women really do benefit by the higher waistlines, shorter rises and pant legs, and small high armholes of petite brands. But since most women are 5'4" or under in the first place, shuttling them off to a separate department or floor as if they're another species is kind of ridiculous. Get into the stylish brands that offer a petite size range and petition your favorite stores to expand the selection range in this category. Check out Ann Taylor Loft, AK Anne Klein, Lauren by Ralph Lauren, Levi's, Calvin Klein, J.Jill, MICHAEL Michael Kors, and Gap.

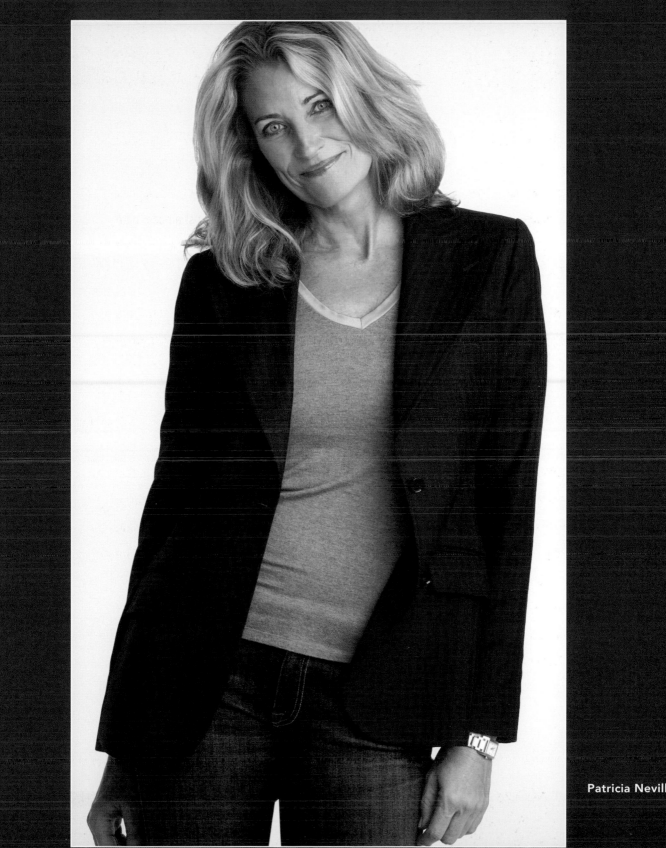

Patricia Nevill

10 Things Women Say About Fashion and What They Really Mean

We're tactful but have ways of getting the message across when asked our opinion. Whether we're shopping together, showing off a new "find," or asking a friend to check out an item we're considering online, there are certain euphemisms we use. Here are our honest thoughts de-coded.

"Not on my watch!"

Don't even think about buying it. If it's already in the closet . . . return! Only a trusted BFF or your mother could say this but pay attention when she does. She means well.

"It's not you."

The truth is it's too tight, too small, and looks like you're trying too hard to look young or thin. It's another way of saying, "Seriously? What are you thinking?"

"Maybe with a great shoe."

This look is too boring, basic, or frumpy. It needs something to lift it out of its misery whether it costs $80 or $650. Next!

"You can do better."

Frankly, you look fat in this.

"See if they have it in another color."

The only thing that could save this would be the color. And then your friend would say, "Love the color. Let's see what else is in that shade."

"It's limiting."

She means that the only place you'd wear this is at home . . . alone.

"You have something like this already."

And *that* looks hideous on you. You can't keep making the same shopping mistake and expect it to work.

"Try sitting."

You have camel-toe and a wedgie. These pants are too tight.

"Let me get you a cardigan."

Check your arms and rear view honey.

"With SPANX, it'll be fine."

Do yourself a favor and try the next size.

CHAPTER EIGHT

CRACKING THE FASHION CODE...TALES FROM THE RACK PACK

Each season designers and stores pretend to come together in one universal mental magic trick and tell us "what's new"—except it really isn't.

Sorry, but there is a lot of fashion BS out there and there's no other way to say it. Every season you'll see lots of extreme looks surface as "the hottest trends." These are the accessories, colors, textures, shapes, and proportions magazines and the media always make a fuss over. They are the ones you see prominently displayed on mannequins, in displays and store windows. There are many reasons this happens and it has nothing to do with the romantic vision of a designer sitting in an atelier draping on a model à la Coco Chanel with just intuition and attitude to guide her.

Dianne Vavra

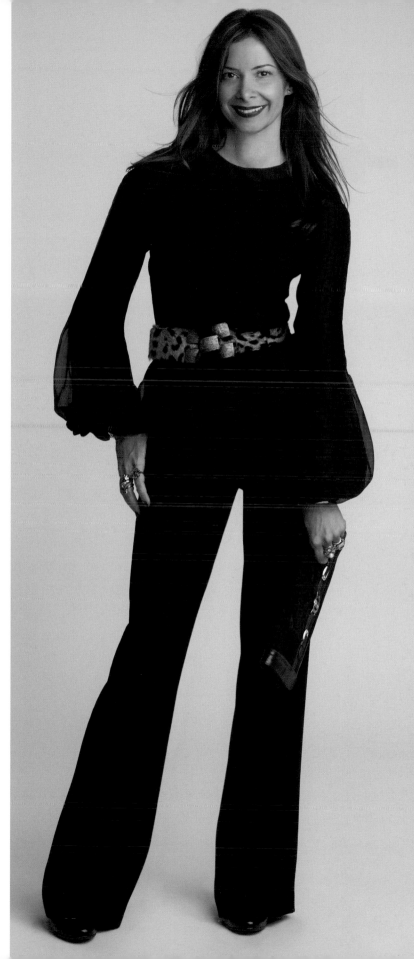

Here's the real backstory

Fashion is a huge industry that relies on other informants for direction now. One of these sources is the fashion forecast field. More inspiration comes from the news media, vintage clothes, and plain old street style. Highly original well-known designers have clear signature looks. Their style comes through in each collection no matter what the seasonal trends are, but more brands (including those well-known labels) are depending on creative teamwork. They need to meet the challenges of a changing economy and demanding knowledgeable consumers like us.

- **Fashion forecasting companies influence style changes.** Designers, retailers, and even some fashion magazines pay forecasters for trend research and analysis. This info sways the runway shows and eventually trickles down to influence the entire mass market of clothes and accessories. The forecast teams hook up clients to global, cultural, technological, and socio-logical trends in music, film, sports, science, TV, art, food, communications, travel, social media, and transportation that will have an impact on how we will live and shop in the year ahead. Although some designers and stores have their own forecasting teams on staff, outside companies provide fast, efficient online info via subscription for anyone.

- **Street style is a major inspiration and urban hipsters offer clues to the next big thing.** This is where grassroots trends like fedoras, graffiti prints, plaid shirts, nerd glasses, messenger bags, and granny boots originated. Mainstream hipster brands like American Apparel and Urban Outfitters get their subculture vibe direct from hipster epicenters like Williamsburg in Brooklyn, downtown NYC, Portland, and Seattle.

- **E-tail and social media fashion sites that provide style suggestions from its users are idea centers for design teams.** These can inspire your own creative mixes although the demo tends to be young. Shopstyle.com for example has a Stylebook component where users create and share their style by mixing and matching items. Refinery29.com covers women with interesting street style via snaps from major cities. Polyvore.com users offer fellow fashion lovers community advice on shopping. Designer teams check these sites regularly for inspiration. Pinterest members reveal online what trends and items attract them too.

- **Vintage stores, consignment shops, and flea markets are scoured for ideas.** True hipsters look for dresses, leather pieces, and accessories at thrift shops, and label hunters seek out vintage designer clothes at consignment shops and online auctions. So do design teams. I know three top women designers well over 40 who practically live at flea and second-hand markets all around the world and it shows up in their use of color, pattern, and accessories.

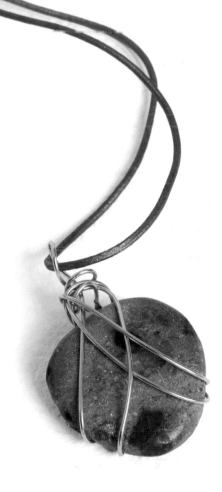

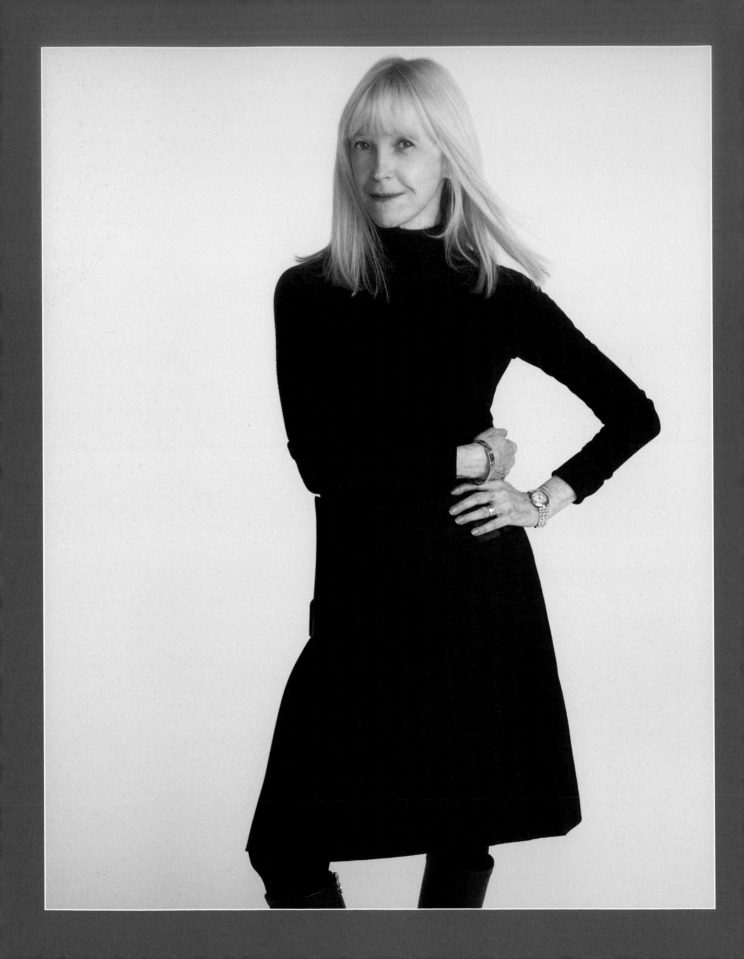

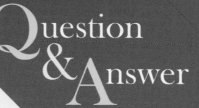

Q: What really influences your fashion purchases now?

A: My lifestyle, my body, my wallet, and trends—in that order. Me too! Same thing! I used to buy way too much. Driven by my job and enthusiasm for fashion I made some great but also quite a few bad choices along the way. My life as a fashion editor for women 40+ was truly on-the-job training since my readers and I shared the same issues. We were aging together. Certain designers always seemed to be reading my mind. Oddly enough they are all women of a certain age now, too, and still going strong. I was an early adapter of Norma Kamali, Diane von Furstenberg, and Donna Karan. Donna's first power suits with nipped waists and draped skirts, shirt-style bodysuits, silk and cashmere pieces, and truly amazing belts simplified my life for a few years. Norma's stretch jersey dresses, down sleeping bag coats and 1940s-inspired swimsuits solved my dress-up, winter, and beach issues. And Diane's black and animal print wrap dresses made travel, business trips, and getting dressed for work at 6 a.m. easy. I still have most of these clothes and they are just as wearable and modern today (I did have the Donna jackets and shoulders altered to be absolutely truthful). When I'm shopping I ask every item these four questions and so should you. Think of it as a fashion audition:

- Do you work for my real life as it is today?
- Do you genuinely flatter my body?
- Can I afford you?
- Do you update or upgrade my wardrobe?

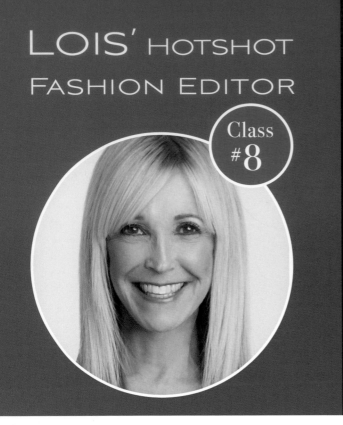

LOIS' HOTSHOT
FASHION EDITOR

Class
#8

10 Ways
Not To Get
Tricked
or Trapped
by Fashion

1. Runway looks are sometimes just for show. Get inspired but don't take it too seriously.

There's a lot of entertainment value in the runway. Shows provide a media circus for new designers, proven designers, and the celebrities who now take up a hefty portion of the first row. This goes way beyond what advertising can do for promotion and let me tell you, advertising is expensive. In just one runway show, a designer gets millions of dollars worth of free PR as the collection is blogged and reported live from the audience. Lots of the looks are more extreme on the runway than those ultimately shipped to stores. Some of these looks never make it to the stores at all. They're deleted from the lineup as buyers place their orders. One of the most irritating behind-the-scenes facts of fashion life is when editors photograph great clothes and have a fact-checking assistant tell you later (as we go to press), "They're not making that after all." Arrrrrrgh!

2. Your timetable and fashion's are not the same. Stick to yours.

Buy in real time whenever possible—that is, when you'll actually be wearing something. Designers and manufacturers are always at least six months ahead of the season we're living in and further ahead than that in their planning. Store buyers are already ordering next spring's clothes during fall when we're just getting into sweaters and tights again. Spring clothes get shipped to stores in February and March. Don't feel pushed into buying too early. First of all, the first markdowns usually start six to eight weeks after an item arrives in the store. Every single store—big or small—has to move inventory on to keep making space for new shipments.

Not all fall/spring/summer/winter clothes arrive at the same time either. Shipments are staggered and the best of the season may not arrive until the second or third shipment. So keep the tags on for returns of items you haven't worn.

3. Stay Skeptical.

When a garment looks too good to be true in a catalog, photo, or online it probably is.

Whether the dress is a $2,000 designer original or an $88 mass-market knock-off, editors and stylists work hard to make sure the fit, shape, and details look even better in the photo than they do in real life. A great model and photographer work together to manipulate the clothes and enhance them. This is why some models and photographers are paid bigger bucks than others. It's always a combo of styling, pose, angle, lighting, fancy pinning, and post-production Photoshop that make a look or item appealing.

When you look at clothes in catalogs, photos, and online be aware of how much of a garment you really see and what you don't. The picture doesn't always tell the whole story. Models pose in a way that shows the best and leaves inferior details out of the camera's eye.

If I see a catalog photo of a model seated at an angle to the camera with her legs crossed and a bag on her lap, I know she's hiding something about the clothes. A pose can emphasize or reinvent the fit or shape of any item of clothing. That's why you never notice in photos that the rise on a certain pair of pants is way too low, or a dress is too snug through the hips and thighs, or the neckline on a sweater is too deep, or that the pockets bulge or hit the hips in the wrong spot—until you try it on. Models, editors, and stylists are masters of disguise.

4. Look harder. Trends recycle but they're never exactly the same.

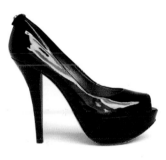

Don't get fooled into thinking vintage items you own are just like the ones on the runway. They may be very similar but something always gives the age away. Whether you're buying a trend for the second time around or just want to recycle a similar oldie back into your wardrobe, check the look of the item and also how it's worn.

Find the news: It may be in shape, proportions, color, print, fabric, or the way things are put together.

Let's say knee-length pencil skirts in bold prints and jellybean colors are a hot trend. They're being shown with chunky shoes and silk blouses. If your "oldie" pencils are neutrals, the color and print part of the trend won't help; the way they're being worn will. Trade your ladylike pumps for peep-toe platforms, wedges, or booties, and your knit tops for blouses (in bold colors or prints), and your skirts slip right into on-trend position.

5. Your new LBD might be orange.

Every season there's a new version of that wardrobe workhorse, the little black dress (aka LBD). We're used to thinking of this as a basic tailored black sheath or shift. Count on every designer to give it a this-season spin. Sometimes designers and editors collectively decree that the new LBD is actually pink or orange or grey. Don't let that throw you but don't rule it out either. The color just might work for you a zillion different ways and wake up your closet, or you might pick up on fresh details and stick to black.

Here's how to shop for a great "LBD" (whatever the color):

Start by selecting a body-skimming style with a knee-length. Look for dresses that are straight and slim, slightly contoured, or A-line. Edit out any that are minis, shapeless, too ruched, or clingy.

Choose matte, seasonless fabrics like lightweight stretch wool, rayon, jersey, or viscose. You want a new LBD to be all around flexible so avoid shine and light silks or dense wools.

Check the neckline. Simple boatnecks, high Vs, and jewel necks are classy. A slight asymmetry in the cut of the neckline, subtle draping, twisting of the fabric, or pleating can add a distinctive look without sabotaging versatility.

Try potential buys with flats and heels. To get a realistic idea of the versatility of any dress, test it with a cardigan or jacket, a belt, and jewelry. See how you can vary the look.

6. Don't get sidetracked by sales racks or flash sales.

This is where we really lose it. Buying items we don't need because they're there and marked down 65 percent is not smart. Occasionally a dress or jacket you've been stalking will turn up, but nine times out of ten it won't be your size. Never buy sale items that are too small thinking you'll diet into them (who needs the stress?) or ones that require major tailoring and a batch of new accessories to work.

Here's when the sales make sense:

To buy luxurious basics to upgrade your everyday life: Anything from cashmere sweaters to pricey bras or the perfect slim pants

To nab a big-ticket seasonal item at the end of a season for next year: Like a fur, winter coat, or cold-weather boots

To get duplicates of specific items you own and love from brands you own and love: The ideal cords, a stack of fresh tees, ballet flats

To upgrade or update your "good" nude and black shoes: Better shoes lift everything you wear.

To buy dressy shoes for evening: This is when to nab sparkly, outrageous pumps and sandals.

7. Take a few risks now when you buy new pieces.

The worst that can happen is you'll make a few mistakes; the best is you might find new ways to wear things or better versions of your same old reliable basics. This is a good way to add variety to your favorite wardrobe colors and freshen your one-color strategy.

For example, if browns and beiges play a major role in your closet you might add slim camel suede boots, a glossy patent leather hobo in copper, or a silk blouse in terracotta and beige stripes.

8. Cultivate a relationship with sales people.

Nine times out of ten sales assistants will say "love your bag" the minute you enter their line of vision. Don't get hooked. This is a smart customer relations gimmick. Look for a salesperson with style similar to your own.

Ask a sneaky question involving stylish celebs to see if it's a good match: "I'm going for a Victoria Beckham/Anna Wintour kind of look—ladylike but modern. What can you suggest?" or "I like bright print dresses with belts like the ones Michelle Obama wears."

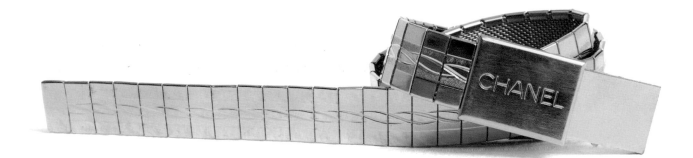

9. Consider new shoes and accessories first.

If these do the trick, you may not want to bother buying clothes. For most women, shoes and bags are an easy update. They quickly change a last-year look to a this-year one. Stores actually like you to buy shoes and bags because accessories provide higher profit margins. This is why shoe and bag departments have grown to take over entire floors in department stores.

Accessories don't all need to match but a team that works together is smart strategy.

Scale matters too. Bags and shoes need to work with your body proportions and clothes. While a sleek clutch looks great with ballet flats, kittens, or slim heels, a big satchel or tote can handle a platform pump or wedge. Mixing it up is what makes style.

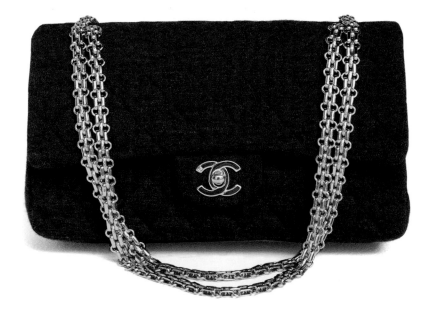

10. Pay attention to your breasts and bras.

After 40, weight changes, health concerns, and genes make their mark. Breast changes affect the fit most, though you probably thought your waist would be the culprit. Hormonal fluctuations and fluid retention can give breasts a puffy or bloated feeling that makes everyday bras, tops, and knits suddenly uncomfortable. If you're over 40 and work out with weights to prevent bone loss, you may notice your back getting broader as you develop muscle. The health benefits outweigh the resulting width across the back but the change will influence your bra size and fit of your clothes. Women who have had reconstructive breast surgery or a mastectomy without a follow-up procedure think differently about clothes too, of course. The crazy thing is all through these changes most of us insist on wearing the same bra size we've worn since college. We're stubborn about this.

Get refitted ASAP since the right bra size solves all kinds of fashion issues.

A full-coverage bra in the correct size eliminates rolls and bra band flab, lifts saggy breasts, and gives you back a midriff and waist. It even improves your posture and body language. But most of all, the right bra size makes wearing tees, knits, sweaters, dresses, and jerseys easy and flattering. Just do it tomorrow. And splurge—a good bra lasts two years max before it loses its benefits.

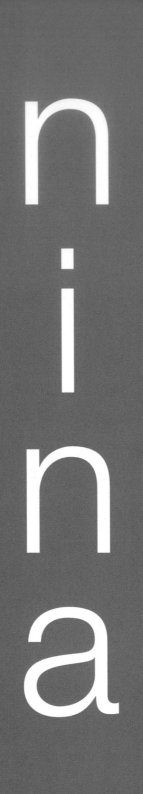

n
i
n
a

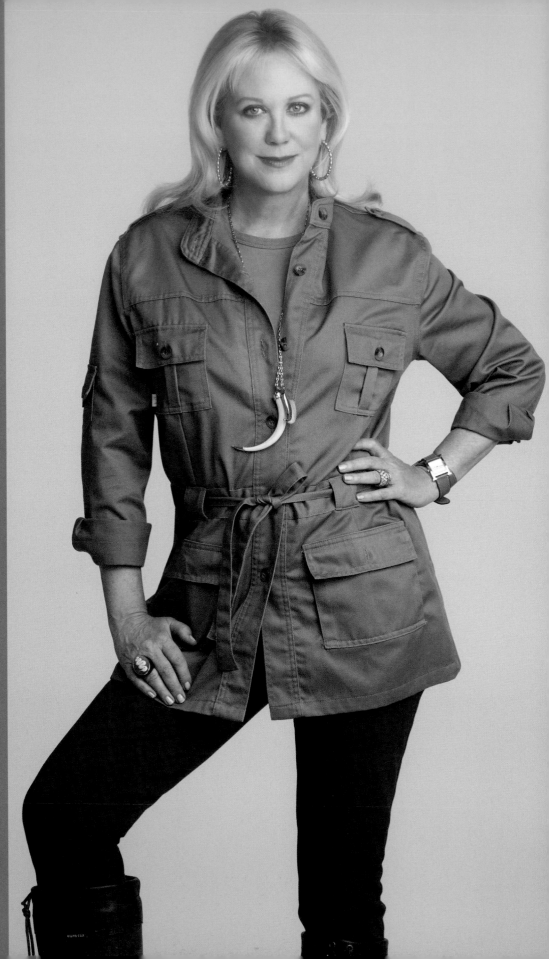

nina on:

age and fashion:

"I believe in age-appropriate clothes but that doesn't mean dowdy or matronly. I wear shortish skirts (not minis) because my legs have held up but try to avoid things that are too tight, too bare, or too short. I have recently decided my arms and back are not as toned as they once were so I have had to re-think what I wear for dressed-up evenings. I have played with different sleeve lengths, which cover the area under the arm and avoid anything that shows too much back. All it takes is knowing your vulnerable spots and finding clever ways to shift the focus with a little fashion camouflage. Wearing one color elongates the body, so do sweaters or jackets that are fingertip length (when you hold your arms straight at your sides). Loading on too many accessories is distracting and aging. I think one great pair of earrings, a cuff, or a wonderful necklace alone is all you need."

nina griscom

Former Ford model, food critic, and lifestyle writer

TRADE SECRETS

GET INTO MEMBERS-ONLY RETAIL SITES.

JOINING RETAIL SITES LIKE GILT GROUPE, IDEELI, MYHABIT, HAUTE LOOK, AND RUELALA CAN NAB YOU DEEP DISCOUNTS. You'll be able to splurge on clothes and accessories from top luxury designers and contemporary brands. They hold flash sales (also called private sales or sample sales) to shop online for a few hours within a specific timeframe for drastically reduced merchandise. This is of course a smart way for retailers and designers to get rid of excess or leftover inventory and move on. If your online site has a Facebook page, you may access alerts to special promotions and unadvertised sales.

LET SHOPPING SITES DO THE HARD WORK.

RESEARCH FASHION SITES LIKE SHOPSTYLE.COM AND POLYVORE.COM DO SOME OF THE EDITING FOR YOU. These sites help you to find exactly what you want fast while staying within your budget and the brands you prefer. They categorize clothes, accessories, and jewelry being sold at a wide variety of retail sites by price, color, brand, item, website, and store. One click immediately links you to the site selling the item. For example, if you're looking for a camel dress in the $100 to $250 range, size 10, the site can find hundreds for you to check out in a matter of seconds. Then you can refine the choices even further by selecting specific designers, a different price range, targeting certain stores, or by how much of a reduction you're seeking from 20 percent to 70 percent off.

SHOP OUTSIDE THE BOX.

TRY SPORTING GOODS STORES, ARMY/NAVY STORES, DEPARTMENTS FOR BOYS, MEN, AND LINGERIE. They're often the best places to find practical fashionable pieces to mix with regular clothes. Fashion editors 40+ love army/navy stores, hunting and fishing shops, sporting goods retailers, and online sites for equestrian clothing. Don't be surprised when you find outerwear jackets, boots, hats, and bags that appear to be the inspiration for a designer trend because they often are. Boys clothes and mens clothes are another offbeat source for women who like a layered look and a fashionable masculine/feminine mix.

I'm always straying into the men's departments at Zara, Gap, J.Crew, and H&M. You'll find luxurious-looking neutral colors like charcoal, indigo, and camel all year long in sweaters, tees, and cardigans, so remember this when the women's market is flooded with pastels and brights. I wear J.Crew mens cotton-cashmere V-neck cardigans in black, navy, charcoal, and brown as layering pieces all year long. Pajamas and loungewear make great layering pieces too so check sales at pricey lingerie departments. Some of those cotton and charmeuse pajama tops make perfect shirts to wear with jeans.

Edris Nichols

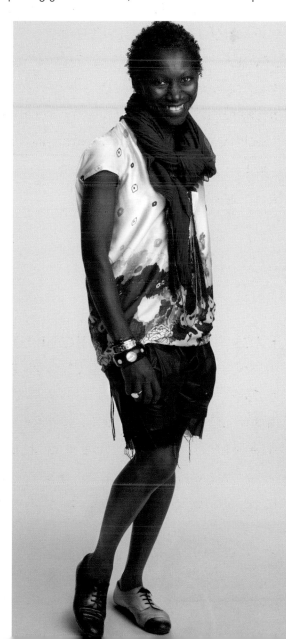

I'm (Still) Obsessed with . . .

Whether you actually buy and wear the clothes by these eight top American designers or ever did is beside the point. The truth is these men and women influenced the way we think about clothes forever. Here are the style tricks you can nab from them.

Calvin Klein

Francisco Costa now designs the brand, but Calvin's clean minimalist message seduces us every time. We love Calvin's underwear but his runway clothes are what really taught us less is more.

Designer trick to borrow: You can be classic but also make it modern and sexy. Choose pared-down sculptural pieces and subtle shades of gray and nude. You don't need pearls, tweeds, red lipstick, and a twinset anymore.

Diane von Furstenberg

Diane changed our world with one wrap-dress in the '70s and came back to do it again in the late '90s, just when we needed her most. She demonstrated how one dress could make us feel feminine, powerful, and sensuous at any age, shape, or size.

Designer trick to borrow: Skip the layers and just wear a jersey wrap dress in a bold, graphic print. It'll give you a waist, tighten your midriff, flatter your bust, camouflage jiggles, and lengthen your body. Add heels and perfume and close the deal.

Certain Designers.

Norma Kamali

Norma taught us a healthy, fit body is the best springboard for leggings and jersey after 40. She made ruching, fleece, and down our everyday favorites.

Designer trick to borrow: Start with a body-hugging base of black stretch jersey and a great pair of sunglasses. To look cozy chic in winter add a shawl-collar down coat with a waist-defining belt; to look sexy and confident in summer swap all except the sunnies for a ruched swimsuit.

Donna Karan

Dressing her body and ours in tailored, urban pieces, Donna became a legend with her brand of reveal and conceal. She taught us womanly curves were an asset, not a hindrance.

Designer trick to borrow: Stop fighting your hourglass shape and use broad, diversionary necklines to balance the body. Always start with a bodysuit, let draping do the camouflaging, and define your waist with a belt.

Michael Kors

Michael showed us all we need to feel like a jet-setter is self-tanner, skinny cargos or white jeans, aviator sunglasses, some double-face cashmere sweaters, and an animal-print bag.

Designer trick to borrow: Keep everything tonal head-to-toe for a chic, uninterrupted silhouette and a luxurious look. Add some gold and a chunky watch and you're done.

Oscar de la Renta

Showed us ladylike style can be flirtatious and contemporary with knee-length uptown dresses in vibrant hothouse colors and jazzy prints.

Designer trick to borrow: Take a perfectly cut body-skimming dress in a femme fatale color like marigold, violet, or a wild floral print, throw on a fitted cropped jacket and colorful heels to match, and you're posh but pretty.

Ralph Lauren

Taught us all that clothes can give anyone a well-bred, old-money look and a romantic, adventurous image through his ads.

Designer trick to borrow: It's all in the masculine/feminine, elegant/sporty mix. Start with a fancy white shirt, add crisp tailored pants or jeans, slip on a jacket in luxurious panne velvet, leather, or cashmere, and you too can look like you have it all.

Tory Burch

This forty-something new kid in the pack endeared herself to us around 2004 with 1960s-inspired blouses, tunics, bags, shirtdresses, and her signature Reva flats.

Designer trick to borrow: Make your basics look cool with vibrant color, geometric prints, and gold accents. Start a new wardrobe strategy of slim tunics and chic flats to wear with leggings or slim cropped pants.

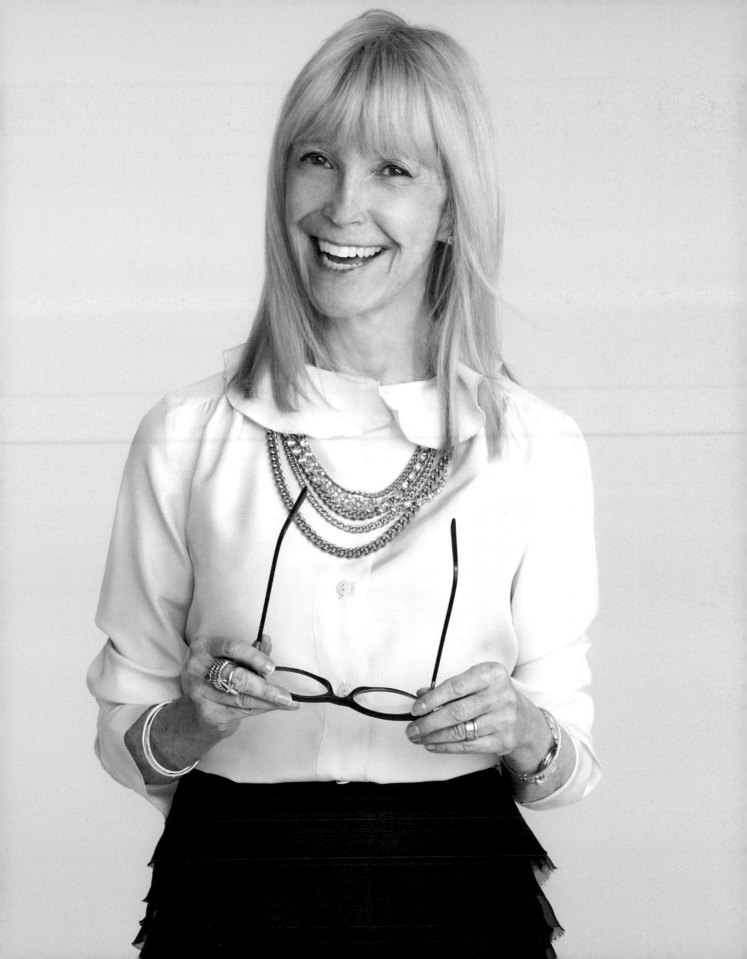

The Best Jewelry For Women 40+ to Buy

Jewelry, real and fake, is a big part of our self-image and personal history. Some of the jewelry we wear is purely emotional and connected to events or moments in our lives. Some of it is trendy or driven by status. But as our bodies and lifestyles shift, certain kinds of jewelry make sense to buy, revive from hibernation, or wear more strategically. Here's the guide to get you there.

Bracelets

There are fashion statement bracelets and I-never-take-them-off bracelets. Fashion-y ones include big cuffs, stacks of bangles, and chunky chain-links. Any of these can be fake, real, or somewhere in between.

Choose cuffs for work. There's no jingling or clinking in meetings, they make a wow impression without the effort of stacking, and look powerful. Because of their size, cuffs don't require additional pieces to make an impact. Wear them on bare skin to accent sleeveless dresses or with a fresh button-down shirt, sleeves pushed up. Try them over long fitted sleeves paired one on either wrist to dress up a basic black sweater.

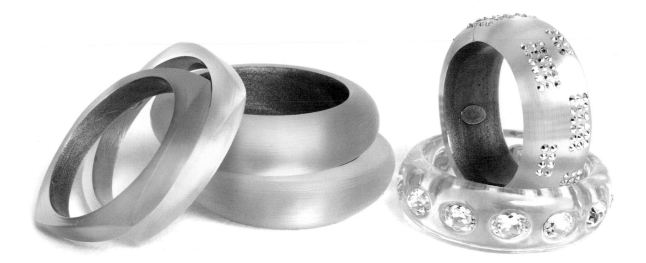

Bangle lovers should collect and stack them as a signature look. Sticking to a single type of bangle—gold, silver, enamel, or resin—gives the stack a more uniform look yet allows you to vary color, width, and texture. They're great for women with long forearms and slim wrists and work as a diversion for those wanting to draw attention away from their upper arms.

Chunky chain link bracelets in gold or silver have a slightly edgy, modern look. Look for shiny, matte, pave links or even link-and-leather combos and feel free to wear several link bracelets together or mix with beaded bracelets and bangles for a more eclectic look. I look for vintage silver plated I.D. bracelets at flea markets and mix them in with dressier costume links and serious silver bangles.

Casual bracelets mixed together add individuality and charisma to anything you wear. Mingle slim chains, tiny jewel-studded slivers, leather wrap bracelets, friendship bracelets, silicone rubber social cause wristbands (to show your support for anything from breast cancer to environmental concerns) and stretchy beaded bracelets. I love to see these personal stacks.

Brooches

Pins go in and out of style and can look cool or dated so be selective. Most women over 40 have worn them at some point and probably have a selection sitting in a shoebox waiting for the trend to hit again. Others have never stopped wearing them.

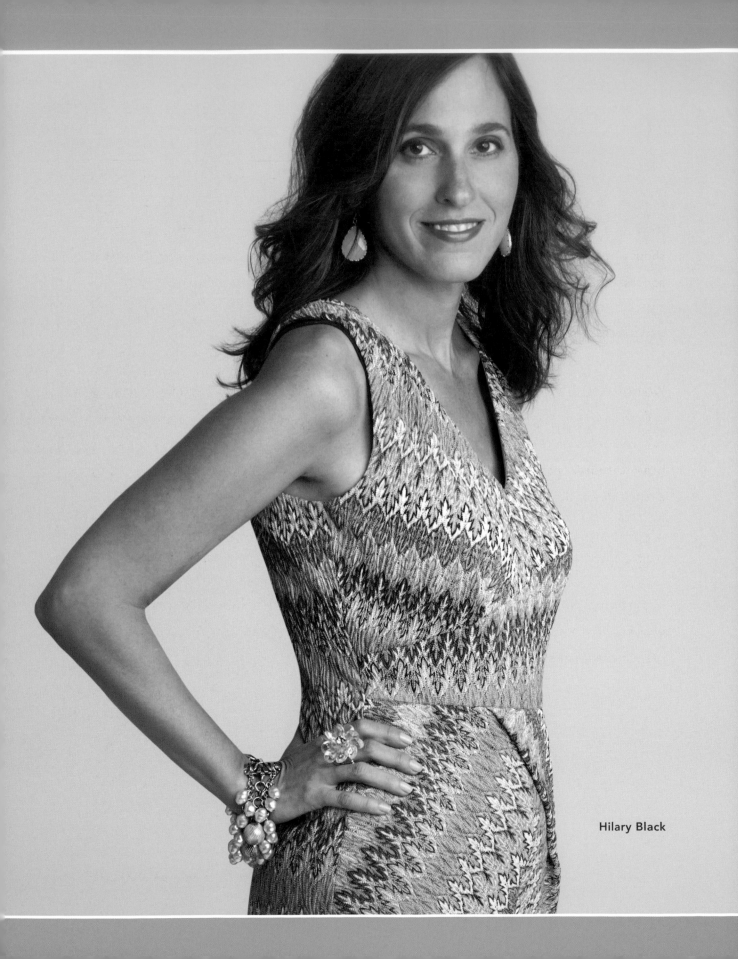

Hilary Black

If you collect and wear brooches, choose a personal theme—animals, flowers, bugs—to give a cluster the most impact.

Worn in unusual places or grouped on a black jacket they can make a powerful statement for work or evening. You can use a brooch or two to close a cardigan, to accent an asymmetric closure on a jacket or a neckline on a dress. One-of-a-kind brooches are great items to snap up at consignment shops and flea markets. I know some women 40+ feel they look "old" and brooches can if worn too seriously and primly on a serious suit, so think creatively.

Earrings

Women after 40 are basically stud wearers or hoop lovers. Fans of big drop earrings eventually realize that a steady diet of heavy earrings makes your piercings droop and stretch aging lobes (which continue to grow forever, like noses) way past the attractive stage. I see loads of droopy lobes with heavy chandelier earrings and it really adds years to your looks. You can have them sewn up by a reputable cosmetic surgeon and then re-pierced when they heal.

At one point women wore big clip-ons to disguise old ears. Statement chandeliers with clips have made a comeback to solve both problems.

Here's my take on multiple piercings and earrings: Make sure you have the haircut and style that goes with lots of studs. I see lots of 40+ women with three or more studs in one ear and a pretty basic, conservative style. It looks off.

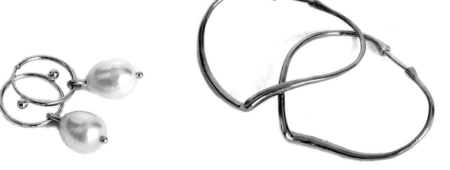

Necklaces

Necklaces after 40 need careful editing because unlike earrings or bracelets they interact directly with your clothes and body. The length, style, and placement require more thought.

Thin delicate chains, pendants, lockets, or charms are more body jewelry than fashion. Whether this is a cross, a tiny heart, or a diamond collarbone grazer, it can be left on under bigger statement necklaces or clothes.

A showy collarbone-length necklace brings attention to your face and peps up tailored dresses, suits, and jackets. Stick to a 16"–18"-length so the emphasis stays high on your chest but look for styles with an adjustable clasp. Then you can customize the fit to nestle lower at the base of your throat or slightly lower to keep your neck long as possible. These chunky shorties are great if you have a large chest or saggy boobs or need an extra shot of glow to ramp up your skin and bring sparkle to your eyes. Isn't that all of us?

Long necklaces work best as a single chain with a wow pendant or amulet to anchor it at the bottom. You can even wear several charms or pendants on the same chain to double up two chains of similar length for more impact. Be careful of any necklace that loops or dangles over the cliff of your boobs in a wide U. It is not going to flatter anything.

Rings

Some women our age stick to a traditional engagement and wedding ring and add a diamond eternity ring as an option. Others mix it up and add other rings to that original stack or wear them on other fingers. There are no rules.

Skinny bands, plain, fancy, studded with stones are the easiest to wear as multiples on the same finger and mixing metals or golds is fine.

I wear two gold Cartier wedding bands stacked on my left hand and a vintage Cartier astrology ring from the Seventies, an eighteenth-century carnelian ring with angels and a gold Bulgari coiled band stacked on my right. Standout cocktail rings are fizzy conversation starters so add these to your evening artillery and be sure you have a manicure.

Watches

A timepiece is one of the things we still wear every day while younger women all seem to check time on their cells. We've been through the gender-neutral bracelet watch craze when everyone was wearing a Rolex, the Swatch and digital trends, and the ladylike revival of slimmer bands and small faces.

The best are classic tanks and over-sized man-style watches.

While pricey brands like Philippe Patek, Audemars Piguet, and Chopard make a major luxury statement, I think the reasonably priced watches by Michael Kors, Marc Jacobs, and Michele make far more sense now for most women. Whether you choose stainless steel, ceramic, gold, or even tortoise or horn (Michael Kors has these), they look smart and are right on the money.

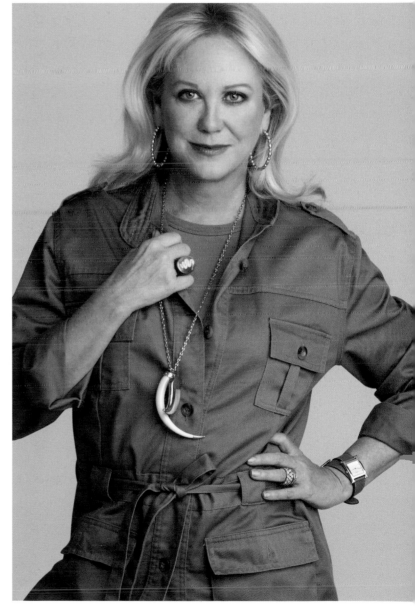

Nina Griscom

The Top Shopping Mistakes Women 40+ Still Make

LET'S ALL STOP BUYING:

Fat boots: The entire point of wearing knee-high leather boots is too slim and elongate your legs. They should be close as possible to the leg in fit, in supple leather, a simple classic shape with a tapered toe. They may be flat or have a heel but their mission is to enhance your legs. Those with a lot of unnecessary hardware, big chunky toes, or oversized platforms and wedges do not.

Jeans that are too distressed or trendy. Jeans are factory-treated to look washed, worn, distressed, and vintage but nothing beats the real thing. Look for any wash you want, any style you prefer from relaxed to skinnies, but skip the faux rips and tears, jeans with rhinestones, decorative trims, or special treatments to look like leather or python. Unless you're actually a rock star they're just plain old cheesy after a certain age.

The same old suits. Look for jackets and pants that do not match or have a fresh feminine shape. If a dress is out of the question try a cropped jacket with a pencil skirt or ankle cropped pants instead of long. Look for soft neutrals or a color instead of black, grey, or pinstripes.

Same old tees. Crew and V-neck tees are classic but pay attention to shape and length, and subtle differences in fit of even basic necklines like these. They get tweaked every year even if you barely notice the changes. Try the new relaxed tees or slightly slouchy ones with a long slim line. They offer body-friendly shaping and subtle camouflage so you can throw out those old oversized ones you've been hanging on to.

Ugly down coats. Walk down any street in New York or Chicago on a winter day and you'll see five hundred down coats, most selected purely for warmth not flattery. You do not want to look like you're wearing the comforter from your bed. The only down coats worth buying (aside from those intended for extreme cold during outdoor sports) have a body-skimming shape or a belt for definition and a big hood or shawl collar that can be flipped up over your head for snow/wind/rain protection. Buy them in black, white, or whatever neutral you wear most. You never have to compromise on style for warmth or vice versa.

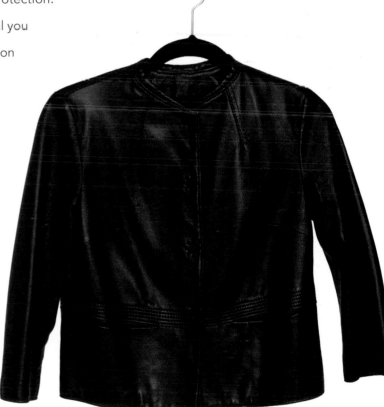

Leather jackets that are too stiff. Leather jackets need to be supple, soft, and fitted or body-skimming. This includes moto/bomber/biker-inspired styles and more feminine cropped jackets. Any leather jacket that feels rigid, stands away from the body, is not pliable, and has a tough look does not belong on your body—no matter who designed it.

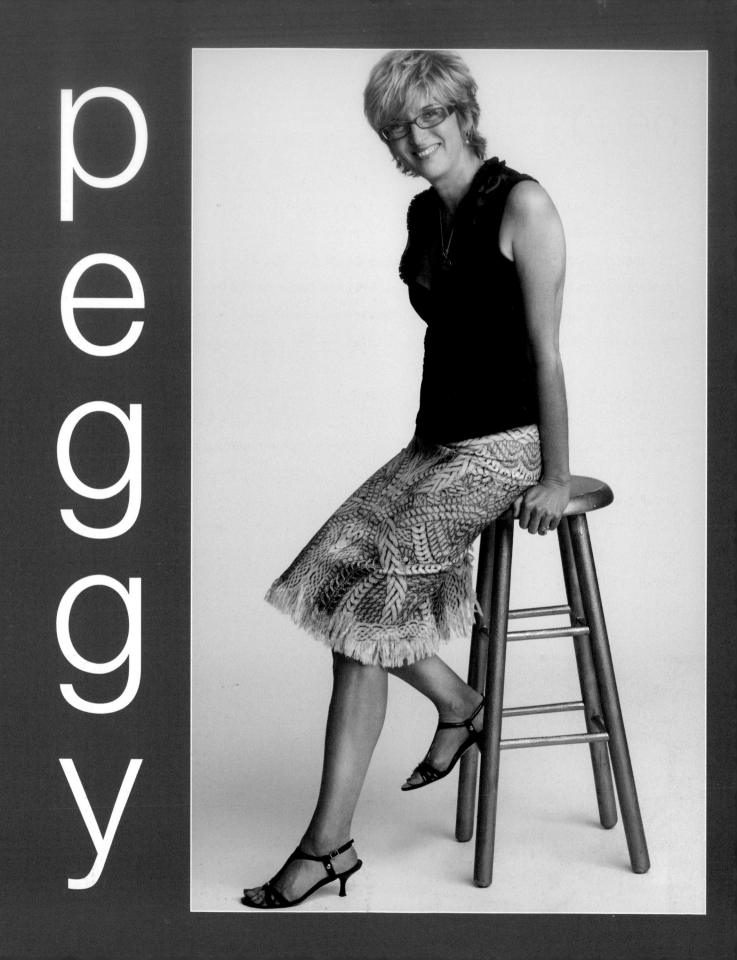

peggy

peggy on:

age and fashion: "I am never going to wear minis again though I don't mind wearing leggings at all. I will also no longer wear clothes that don't make me feel great or shoes that hurt after two blocks. What's really changed is my choice of shoes. I'm constantly looking for the perfect non-old lady shoes that have some sort of padding for comfort. I think super-short or super-tight clothes look inappropriate on older women but then I don't like them on younger women either! I'm conscious of the wear and tear on my joints from carrying big heavy bags so usually I carry two—a small one and a light tote."

style: "I'm trying to be a little edgy yet mostly comfortable. I hate to look like I'm trying too hard. I try to achieve a certain unfussy polish, so certain favorites work for me: separates, jackets, skinny pants, pencil skirts, and flat boots. Nipped-in, closely tailored shirts or jackets give me a waist (without feeling like I have to suck in my stomach) and fishtail pencils that are narrow but have a slight flip at the hem add subtle curves. The Alexander McQueen one I'm wearing here is a good example. I was thrilled when J.Crew started making skinny, flat-front skirts similar to the pricey ones from Prada that I'd fallen in love with. Buying very expensive clothes these days makes me anxious; I feel like I'm stealing from my future old-lady self. Luckily, there are plenty of options out there!"

peggy northrop

Editorial consultant, former editor-in-chief of *MORE* magazine, and editorial director of *Reader's Digest*

Thank You!
XXOO from Lois

To my amazing photographer, **Michael Waring**, who really knows how to make women 40+ look great and feel like Kate Moss. Your lighting, wit, patience, and skill make Botox, fillers, and cosmetic surgery unnecessary.

To the gorgeous women—my friends and colleagues—who shared their style, shopping wisdom, and fashion experience with me and women everywhere: **Annemarie Iverson**, **Cynde Watson**, **Dianne Vavra**, **Edris Nicholls**, **Eve Feuer**, **Felicia Milewicz**, **Gloria Appel**, **Hilary Black**, **Jane Larkworthy**, **Jean Hoehn Zimmerman**, **Jo Gaynor**, **Marilyn Glass**, **Nina Griscom**, **Nikki Wang**, **Patricia Neville**, **Peggy Northrop**, **Valerie Lynn**, and **Valerie Monroe**.

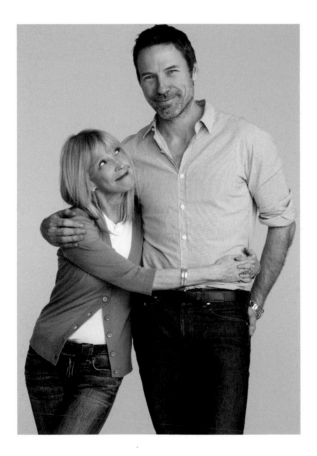

To supermodel **Cheryl Tiegs** for writing the foreword and inspiring our entire generation to smile, feel confident in a swimsuit, and wear everything from jeans to an evening gown fearlessly and with style.

To all at **Location 05 on Hudson Street** for super-smooth shoot days.

To everyone at **Shoot Digital** for making the cover shoot a breeze—and **Hector Tirado** for on-set support and lattes and smoothies.

To our studio pros: **Alexander Yerks** for digital skills, **Evan Y. Lee** for taking a great photo of Michael and I (not easy).

To **Michelle White**, our fantastic retoucher. We all adore you.

Lois and photographer Michael Waring

To makeup guru **Julie Tussey** and hairstylist **Nicole Blais** for making me look so great on the cover and for hours of great girl chat.

To stylist and chum **Suzanne Martine** for cover shoot assistance and cheer.

To makeup and hair pro **Nikki Wang** for making all the real women photographed for this book look glowing and glam on set.

To **Jessica Goico** and my niece **Zoey Wilensky** for assisting on the "model" shoots.

To **Running Press**, my brilliant editor **Cindy De La Hoz**, and talented book designer **Corinda Cook** for making this book a reality.

To my wonderful agent and friend, **Alice Martell**, for legal advice, patience, and always answering my emails—even from vacation.

To my hair team: guru/colorist **Brad Johns** for turning on the lights and keeping me buttery blonde forever and my hairstylist, **Chris Cusano**, for talking me out of growing out my bangs every single month of my life.

To **Susan Duffy** and **Karen Ferko** at Stuart Weitzman for love and shoes!

To my daughters, **Jennifer Jolie** and **Alexandra Jade**, for shopping with me for decades and taking my advice—even now.

To my husband, **Robert Kadanoff**, for his daily fashion dilemmas, love, and support and for hardly ever complaining about my passion for beauty and fashion—or my twenty-three-hours-a-day computer lifestyle.

To my Yorkie-Poo, **Louie**, for unconditional love and feedback on copy read aloud.

To all my super-smart female friends in the beauty, fashion, and publishing industry who pushed and prompted, backed and boosted, encouraged, and egged me on for thirty years in my career as a top beauty and fashion editor: **Myrna Blyth** (publishing legend and my mentor), **Andrea Quinn Robinson** (beauty exec and editor extraordinaire, who got me into this business in the first place), **Susan Duffy** (beauty and fashion PR and marketing genius and confidante),

Charla Krupp (miss you babe), **fashion gurus** Norma Kamali, Carolina Herrera, Lauren Hutton, Betsey Johnson, Nicole Miller, Donna Karan, Adrienne Landau, Christiane Celle, Josie Natori, Adrienne Vittadini, Diane Von Furstenberg, Kate Spade, Tory Burch, Eileen Fisher, Vera Wang, Gabrielle Sanchez, Heidi Weisel, and Selima Salaun. **Beauty chums** Anastasia Soare, Bobbi Brown, Sandy Linter, Karen Kawahara, Sonia Kashuk, Jeanine Lobell, Deborah Lippmann, Mally Roncal, Trish McEvoy, Suzi Weiss Fischmann, Sally Hershberger, Jean and Jane Ford, Essie Weingarten, and Terri de Gunzberg. XXOO

To all the women I've interviewed and worked with on shoots who passed along a fashion tip or trick including: Alana Stewart, Ali MacGraw, Andie MacDowell, Anne Archer, Ann Curry, Rosanna Arquette, B. Smith, Beverly Johnson, Candace Bushnell, Blythe Danner, Bebe Neuwirth, Bernadette Peters, Barbara Walters, Carly Simon, Carol Alt, Cher, Christine Ebersole, Christie Brinkley, Christine Baranski, Cybill Shepherd, Deborah Harry, Diane Keaton, Dolly Parton, Elle MacPherson, Ellen Barkin, Fran Drescher, Iman, Ivana Trump, Jacqueline Bisset, Jamie Lee Curtis, Jane Fonda, Jennifer Beals, Jerry Hall, Joan Allen, Joan Collins, Joan Rivers, Jodi Foster, Kathie Lee Gifford, Katie Couric, Kim Cattrall, Linda Evans, Marg Helgenberger, Mariel Hemingway, Marilu Henner, Marisa Berenson, Marla Maples, Marlo Thomas, Mary Steenburgen, Meredith Vieira, Michelle Phillips, Morgan Fairchild, Oprah Winfrey, Peggy Fleming, Peggy Lipton, Phyllis George, Priscilla Presley, Rosanna Arquette, Rosanna Scotto, Sally Field, Shari Belafonte, Sharon Stone, Sigourney Weaver, Susan Lucci, Suzanne Somers, Sonja Braga, Twiggy, and Vanessa Williams. XXOO

To the models who helped me redefine what 40+ looks like and change the attitudes of the beauty and fashion world forever: Patti Hansen, Christie Brinkley, Paulina Porizkova, Janice Dickinson, Isabella Rossellini, Dayle Haddon, Susan Forristal, Nancy Donahue, Kim Alexis, Alva Chinn, Emme Aronson, Julie Wolfe, Veronica Webb, Karen Bjornson, Susan McGraw, Cindy Joseph, Dianne Dewitt, Lisa Berkley, Karen Graham, Susan Hess, Lara Harris, Grethe Holby, Vendela, Jane Powers, Louise Vyent, Penni B., Cheri LaRocque, Cecelia Rodhe, Lois Chiles, Donna Bunte, Rosie Vela, Isabelle Townsend, Michelle Stevens, Gunilla Lindblad, and Pat Tracey. XXOO

And to all the millions of women 40+ who read my magazine features, columns, blogs, and books and continue to inspire me every day. You've still got it!!